SEX POSITION COLORING BOOK

Playtime for Couples

Amorata Press

Copyright concept and design © 2013 Ulysses Press and its licensors. All Rights Reserved. Any unauthorized duplication in whole or in part or dissemination of this edition by any means (including but not limited to photocopying, electronic devices, digital versions, and the Internet) will be prosecuted to the fullest extent of the law.

Published by:
Amorata Press
an imprint of Ulysses Press
P.O. Box 3440
Berkeley, CA 94703
www.amoratapress.com

A Hollan Publishing, Inc. Concept

ISBN: 978-1-61243-240-3

Printed in the United States by United Graphics, Inc.

10 9 8 7 6 5 4 3 2 1

Acquisitions editor: Keith Riegert
Managing editor: Claire Chun
Cover Design: Jake Flaherty
Cover illustration: Hollan Publishing
Sex position illustrations: Hollan Publishing
Design and layout: Jake Flaherty
Illustrations: see page 104

Distributed by Publishers Group West

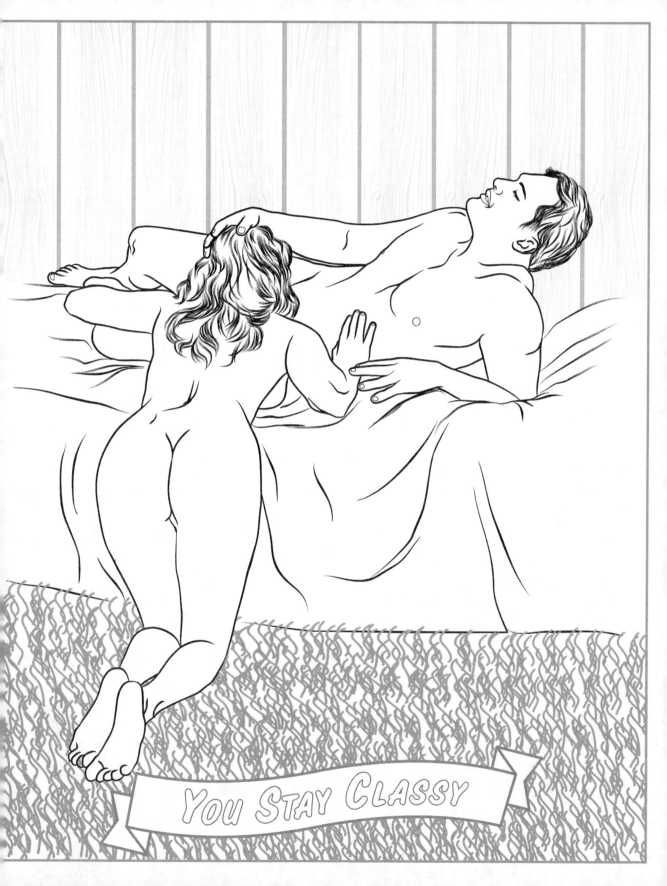

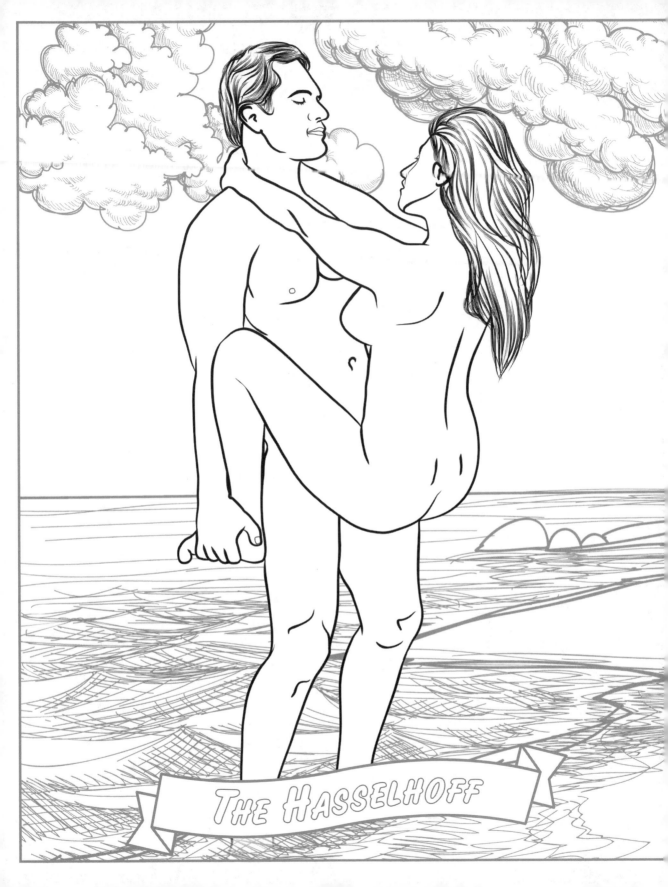

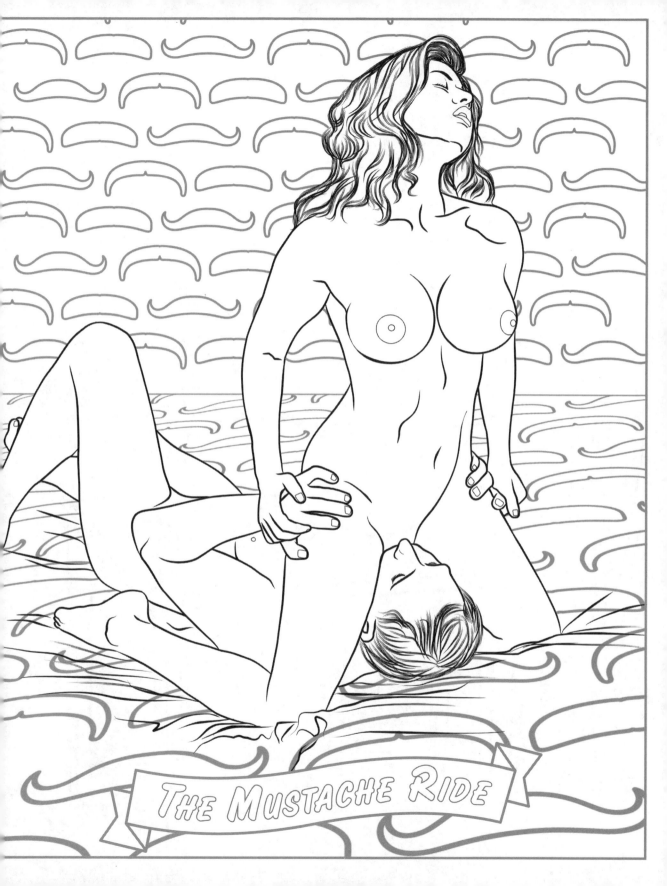

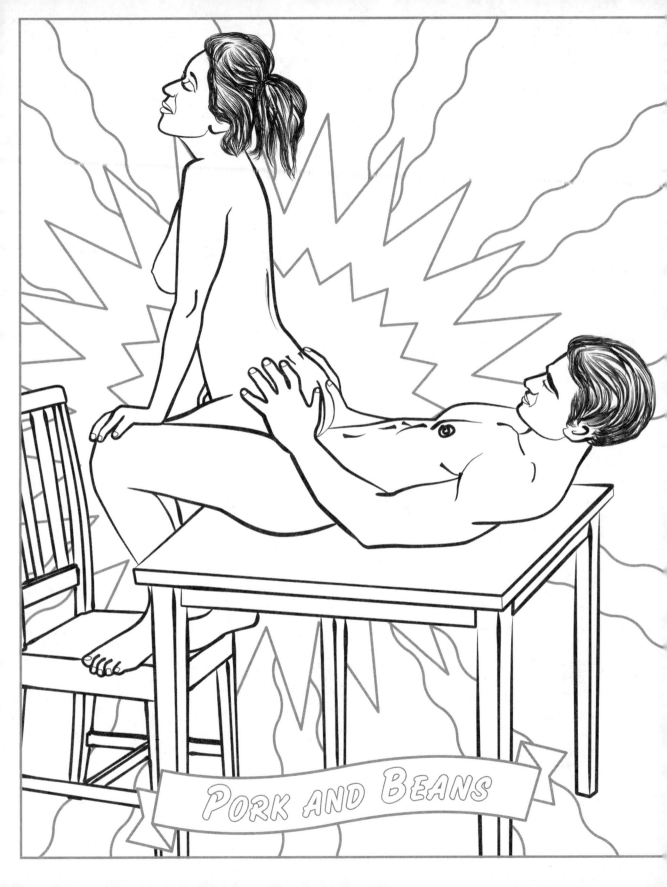

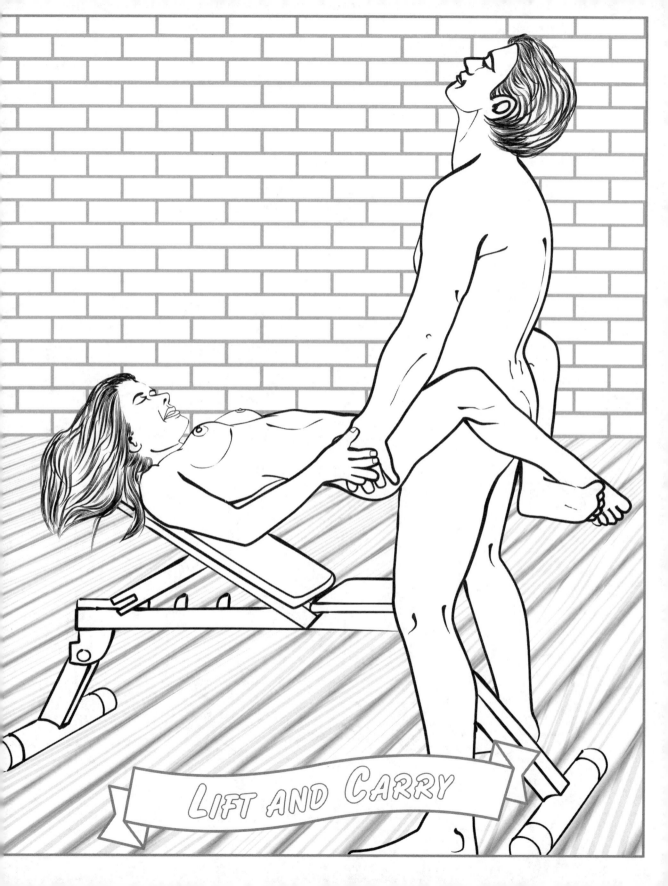

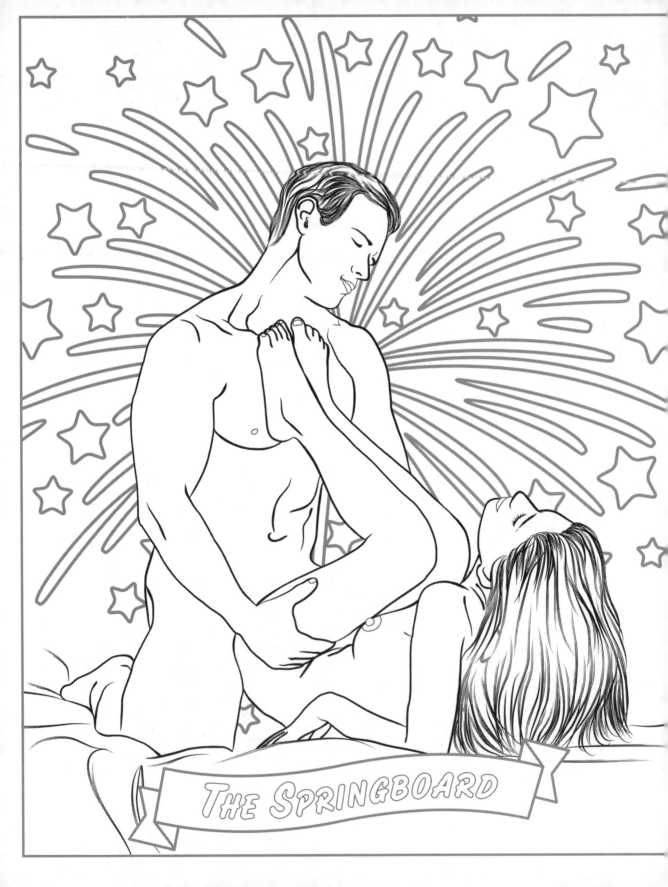

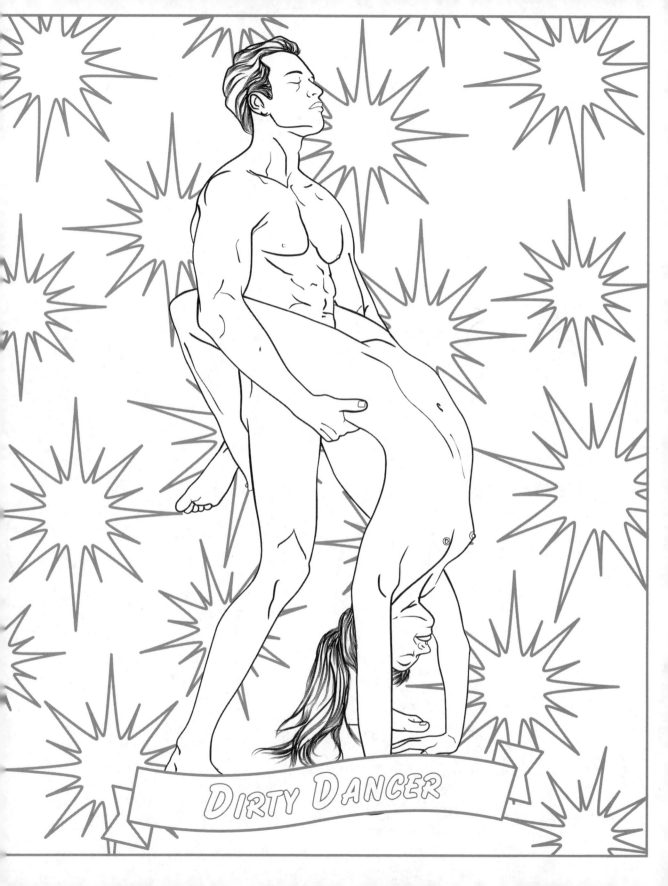

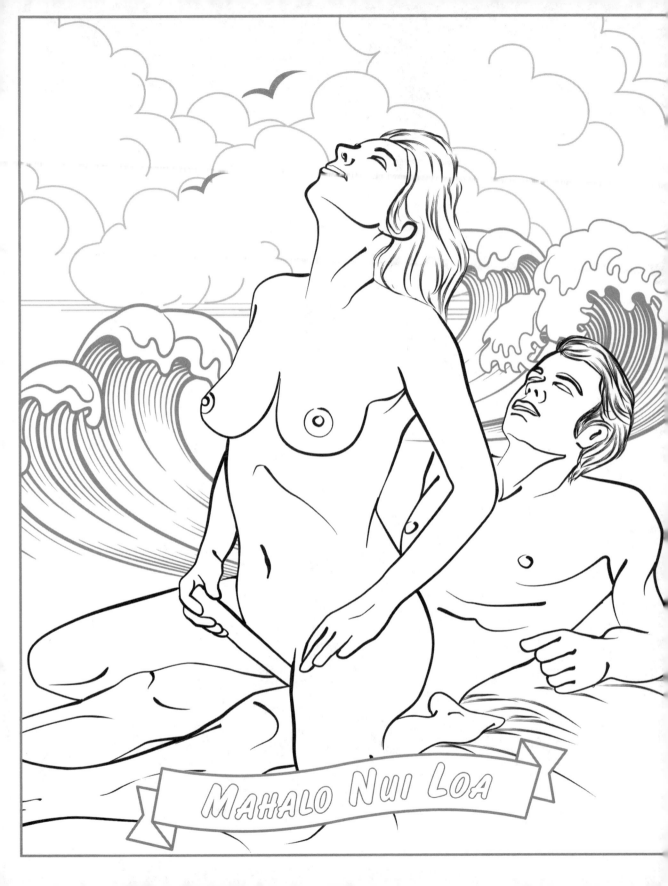

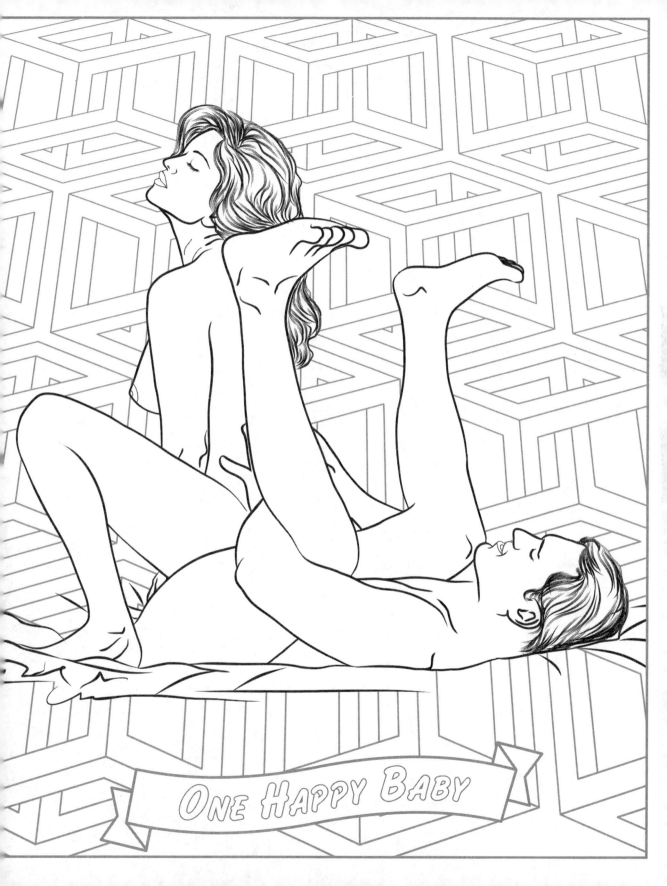

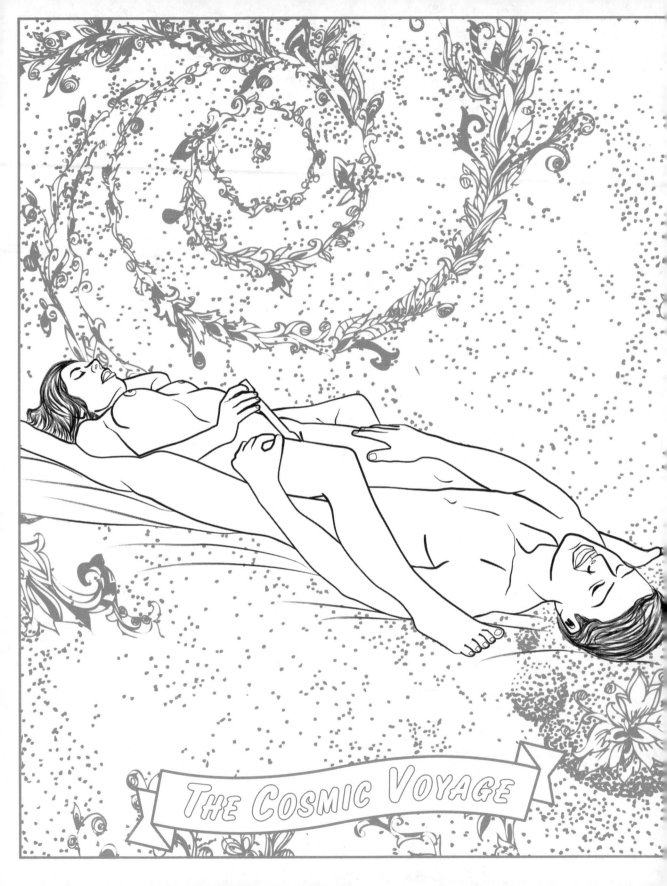

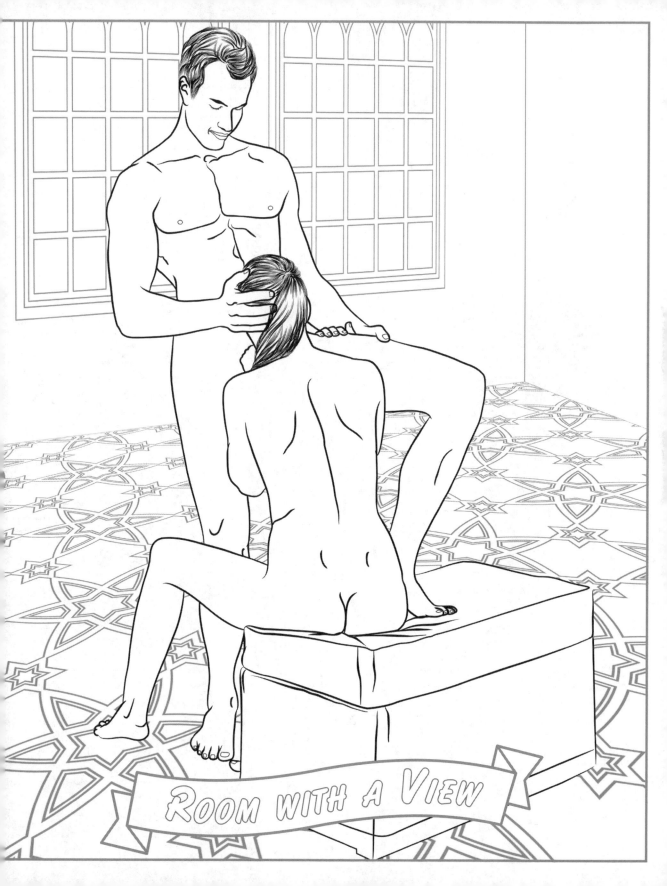

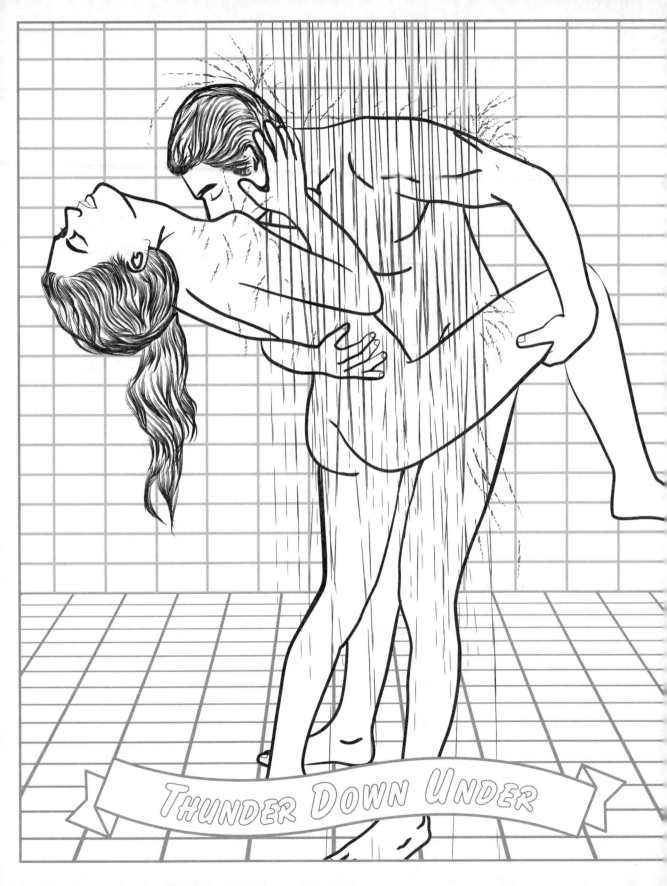

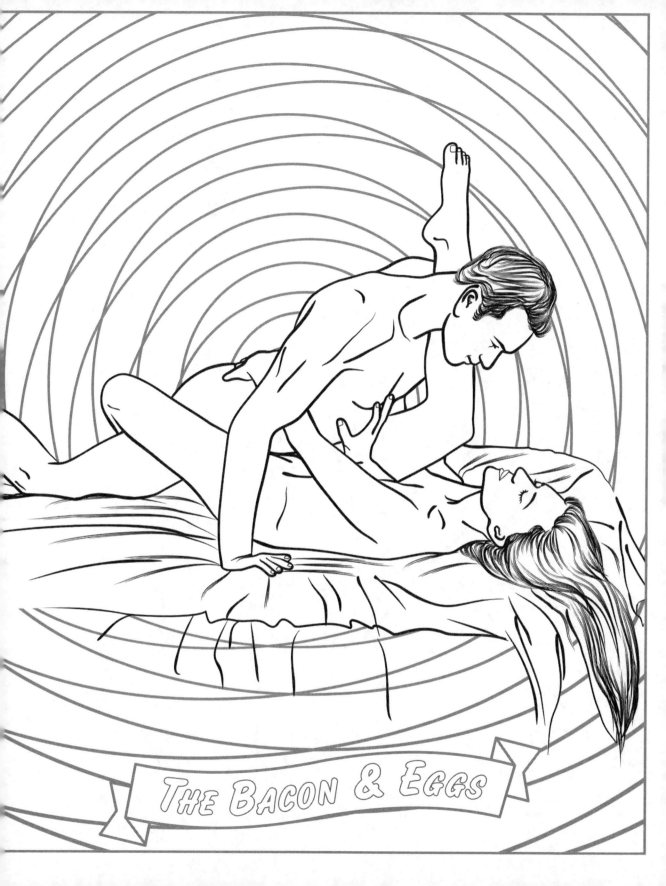

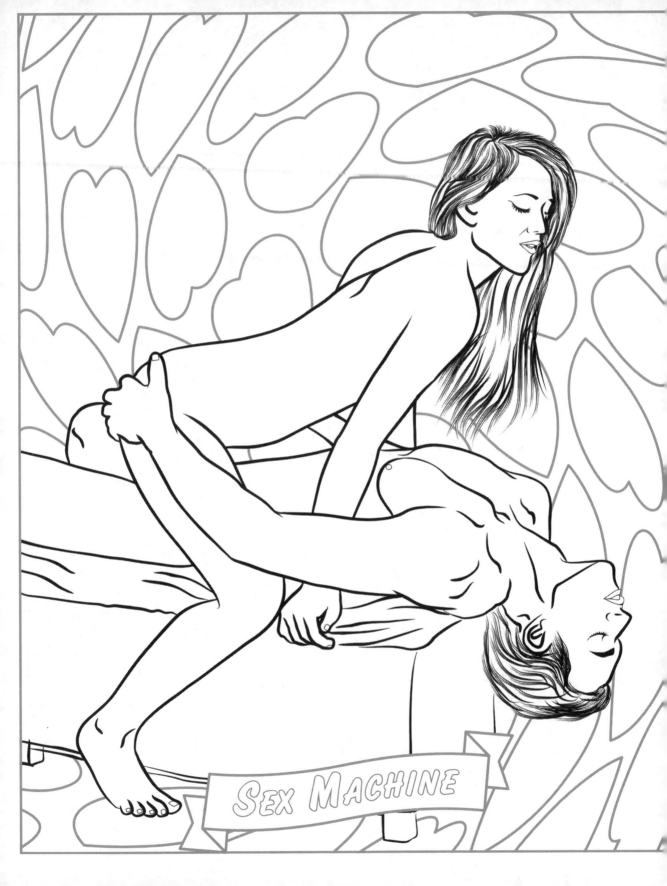

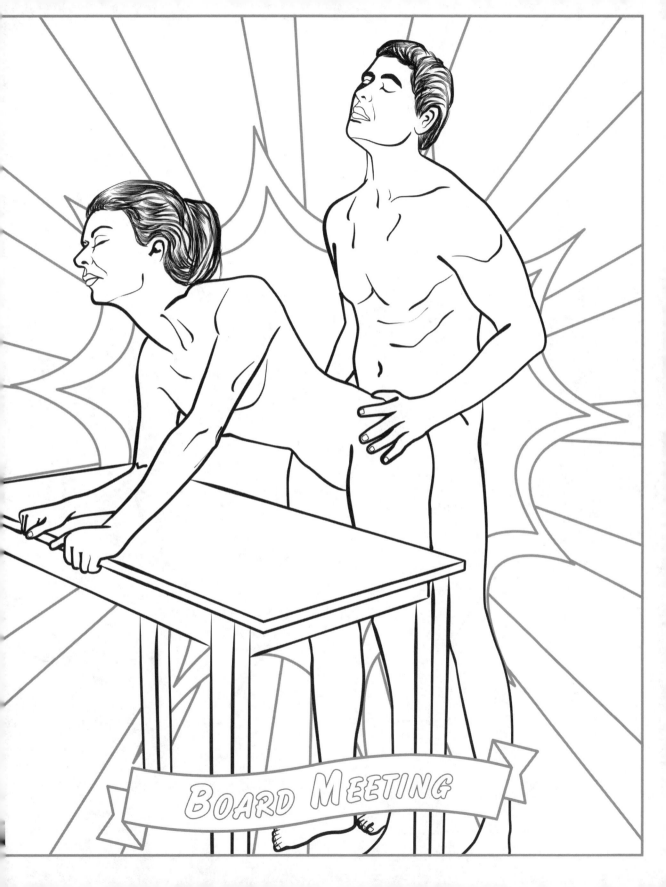

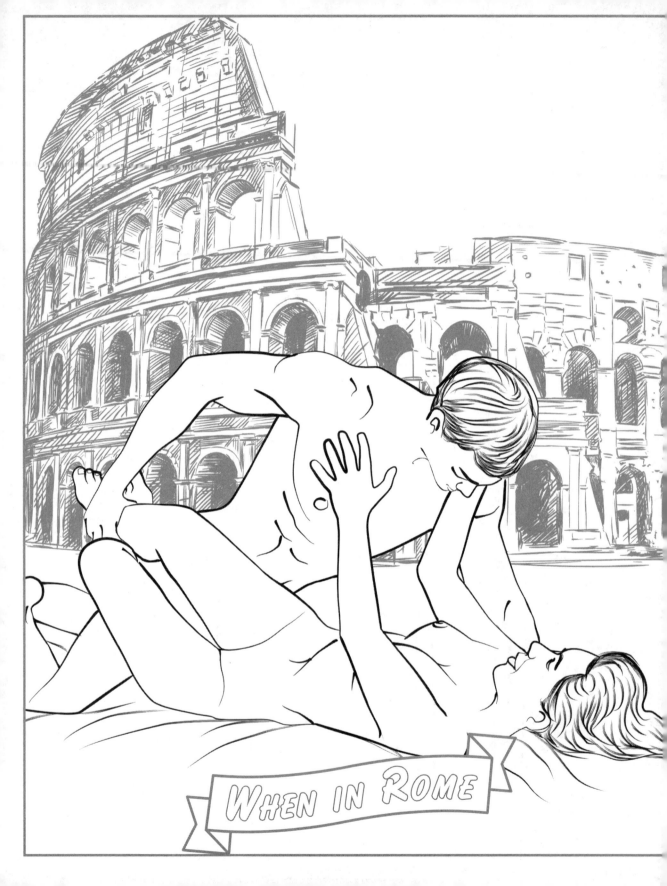

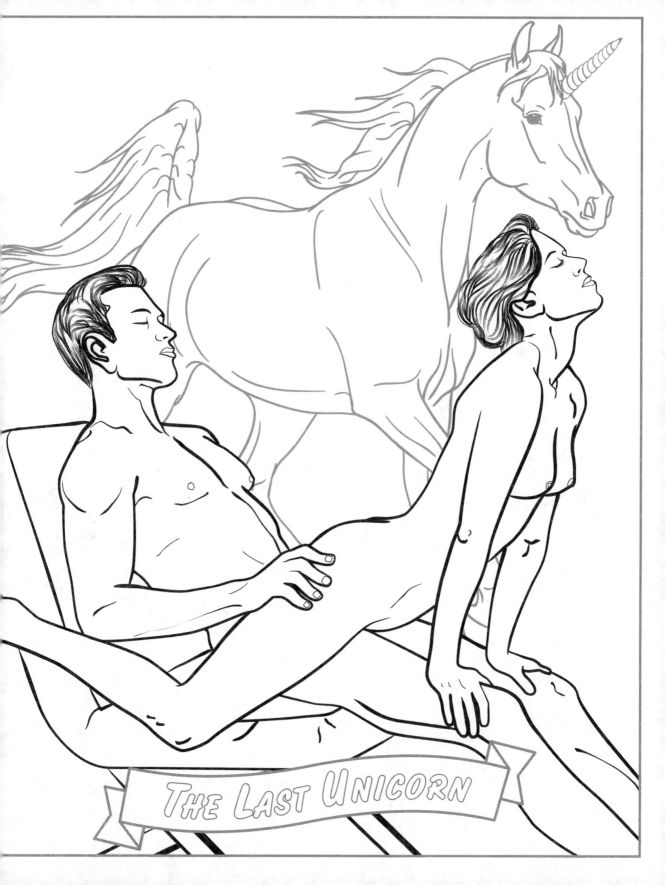

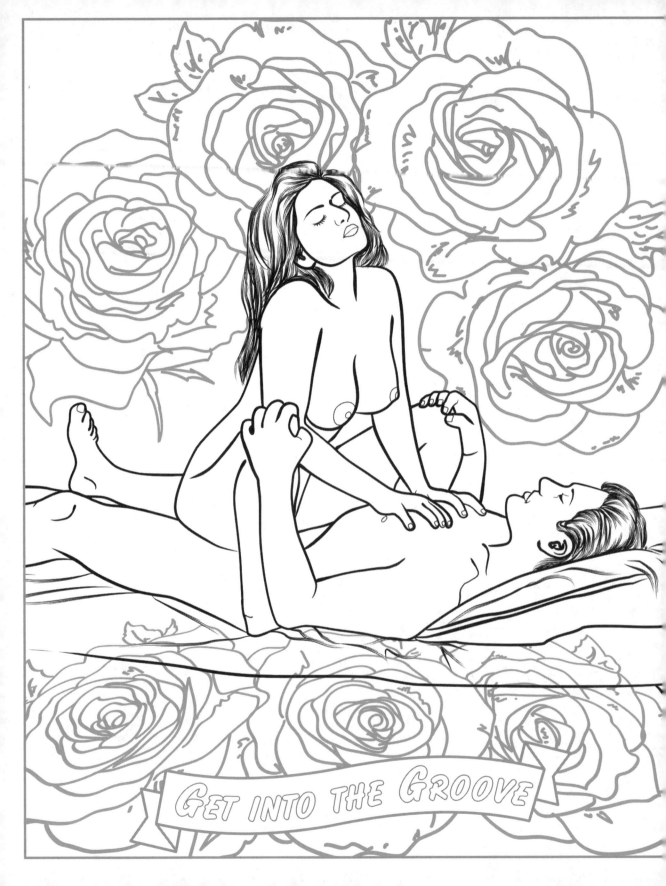

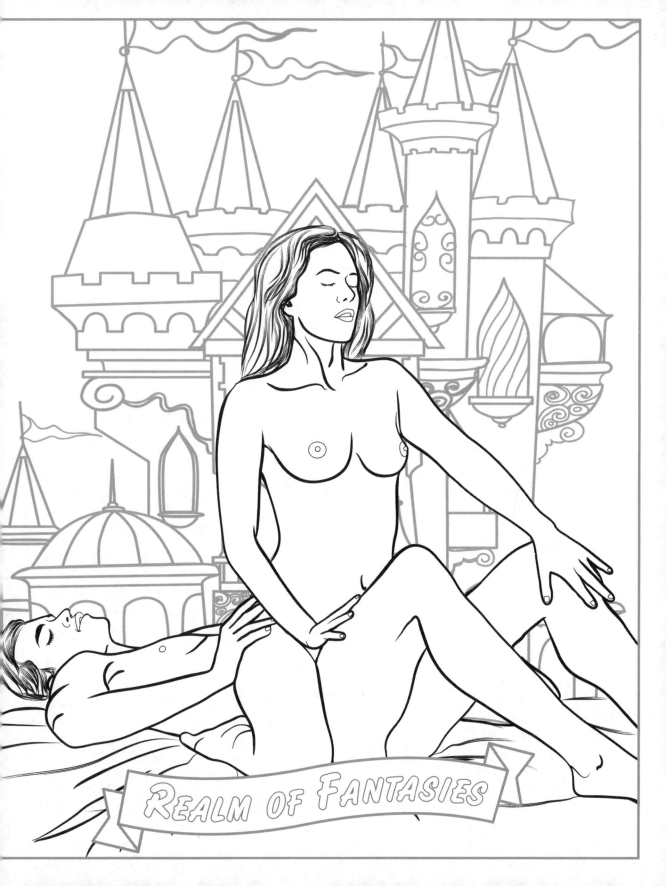

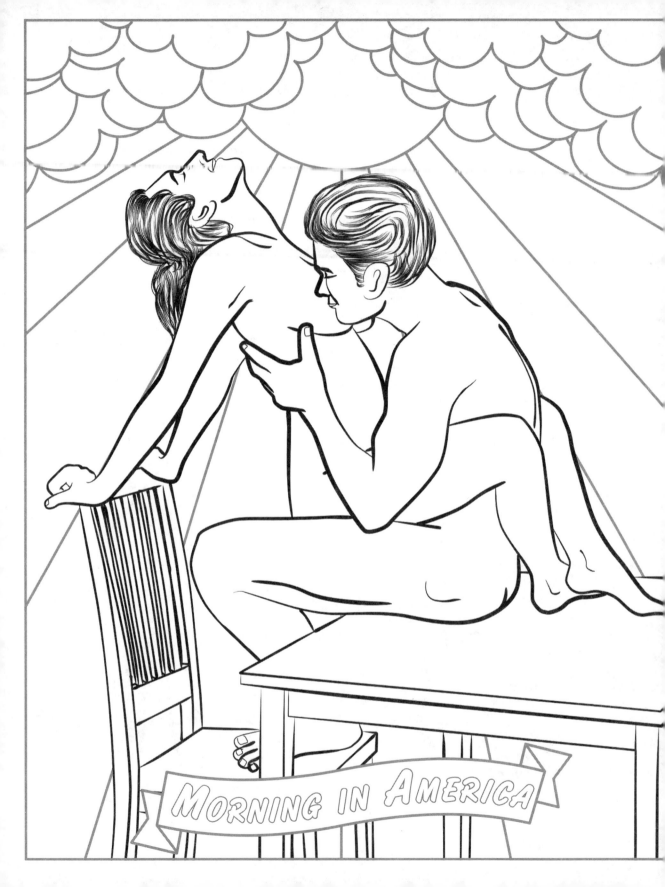

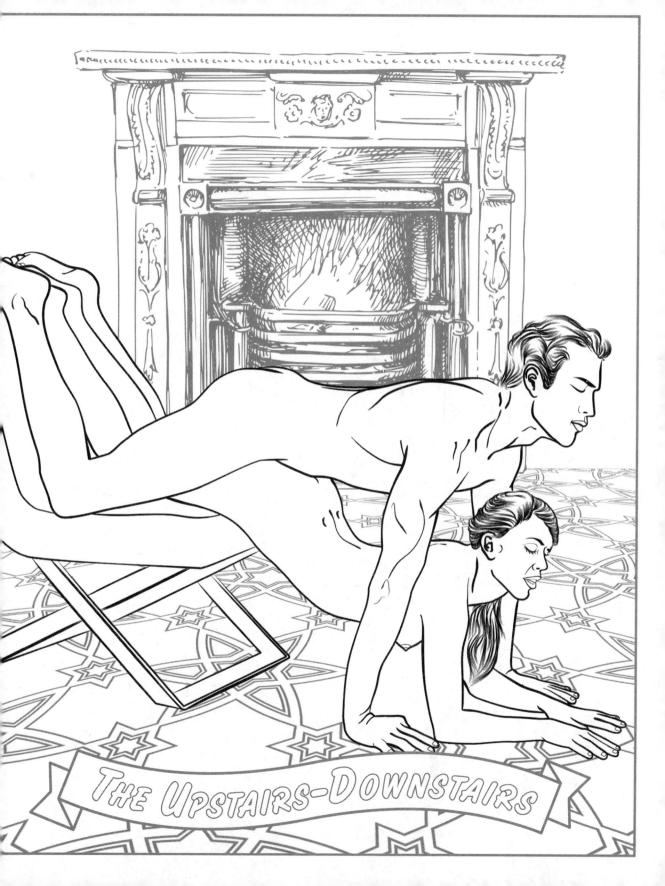

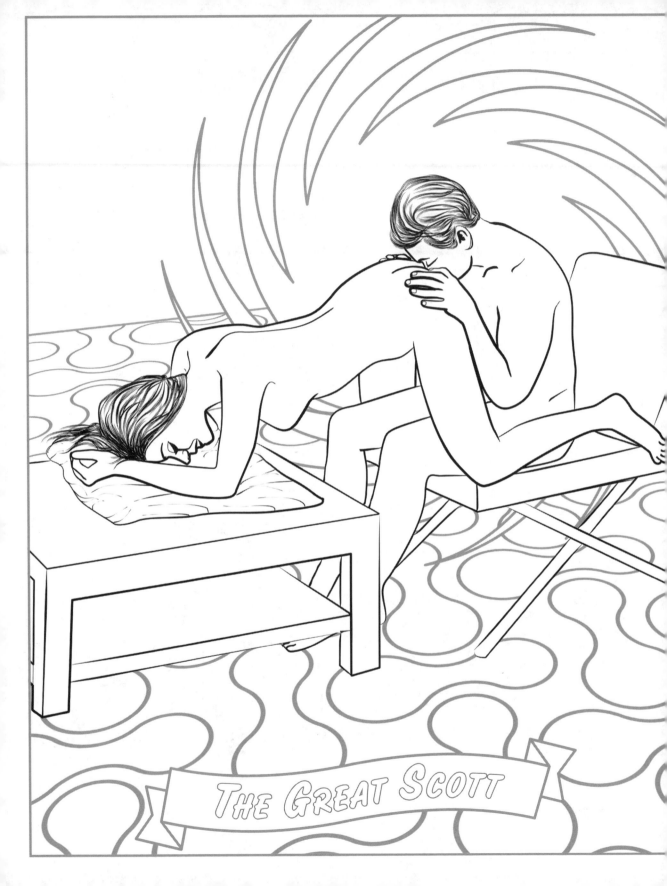

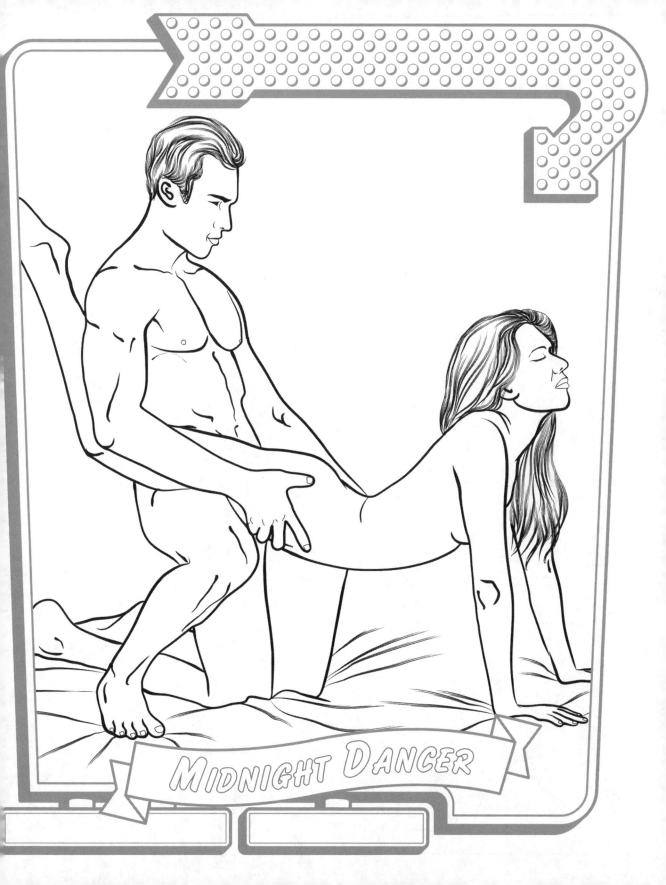

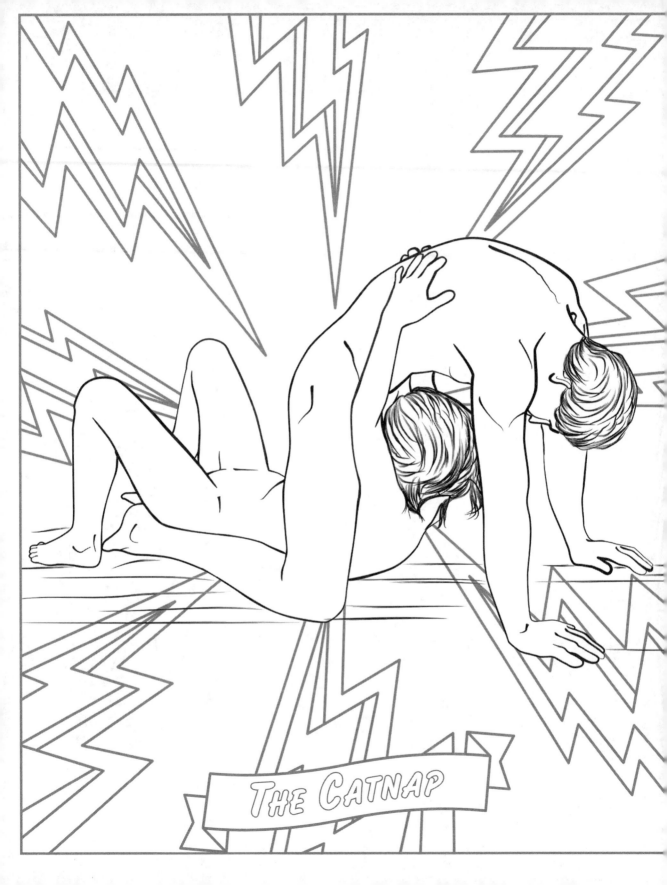

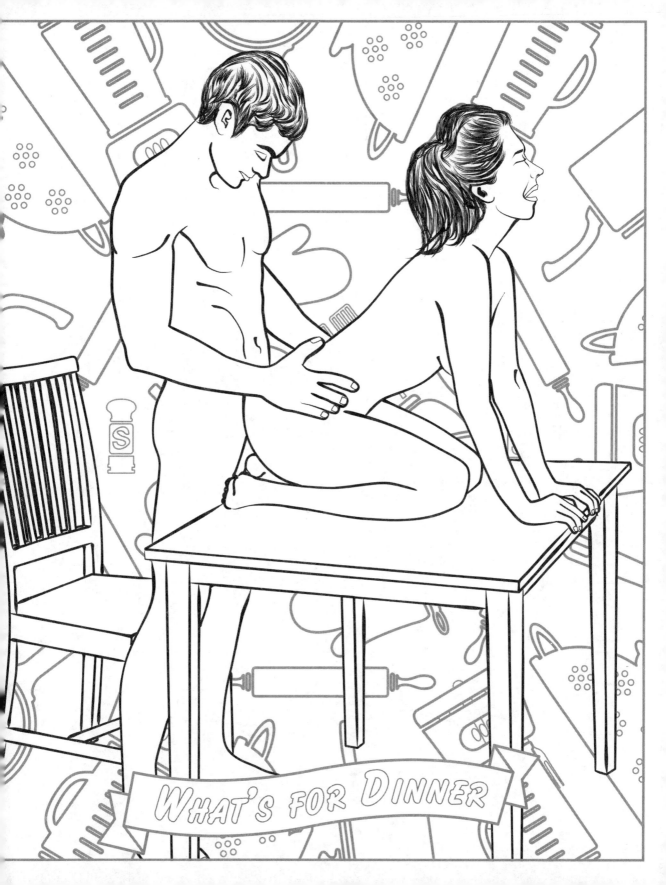

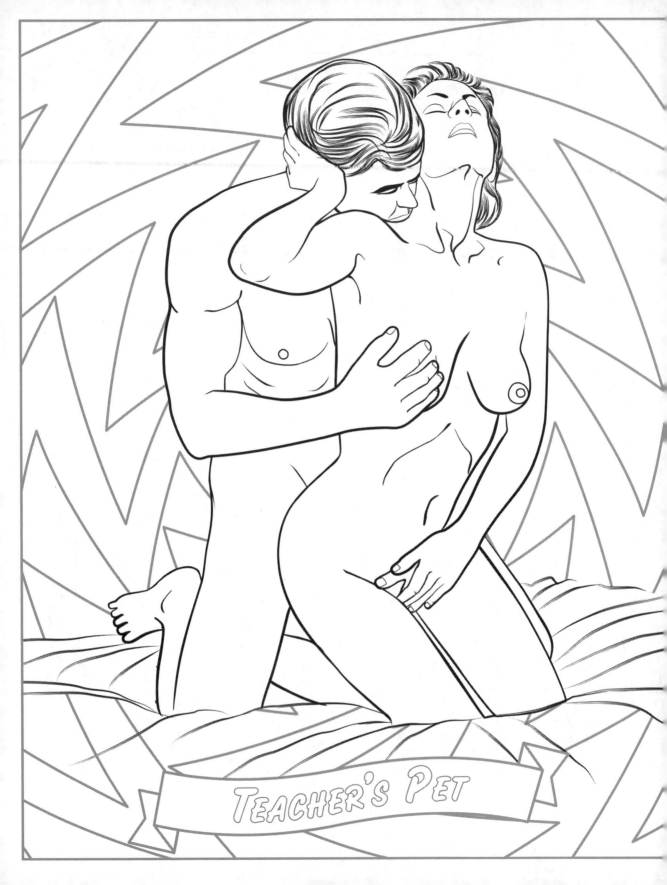

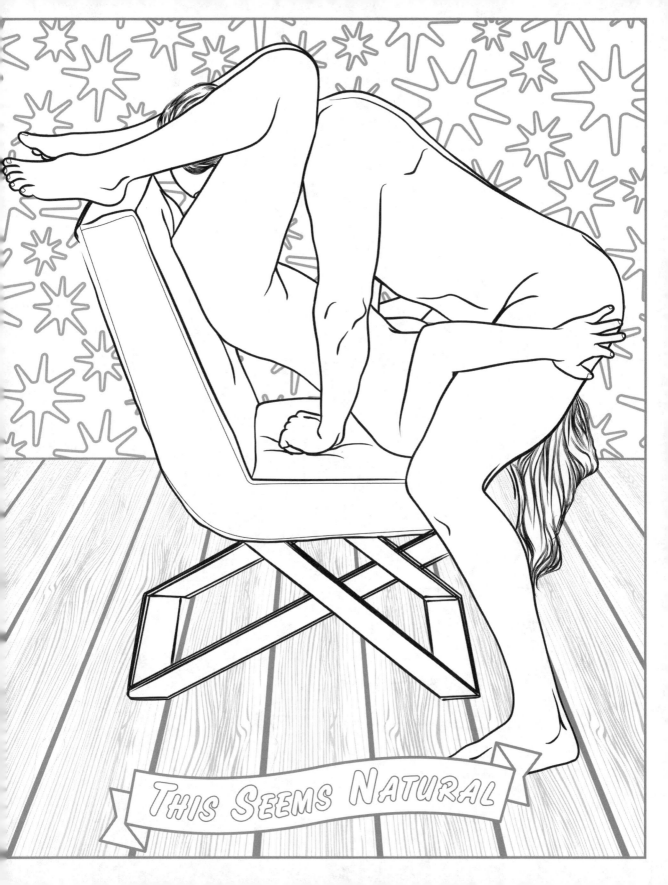

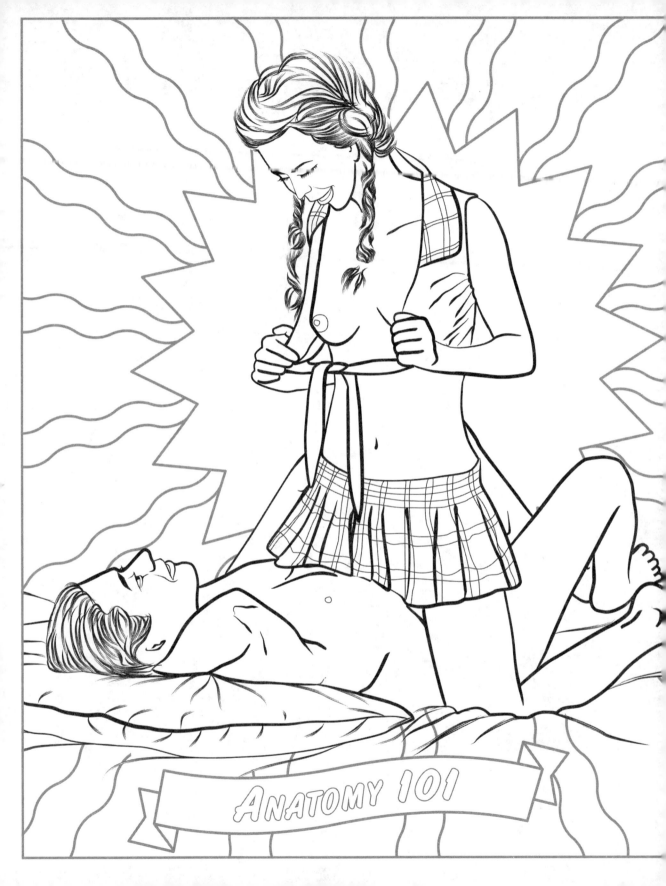

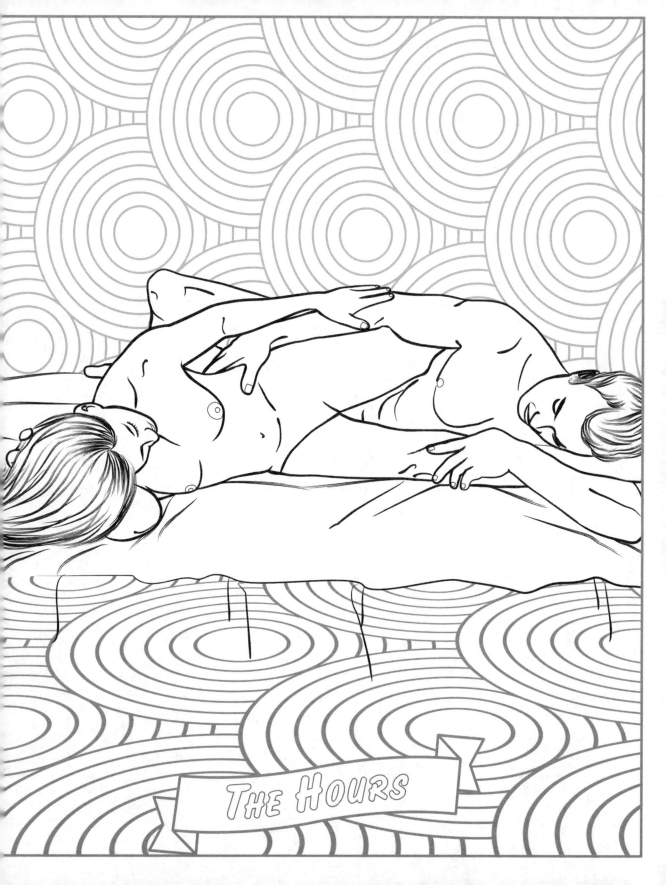

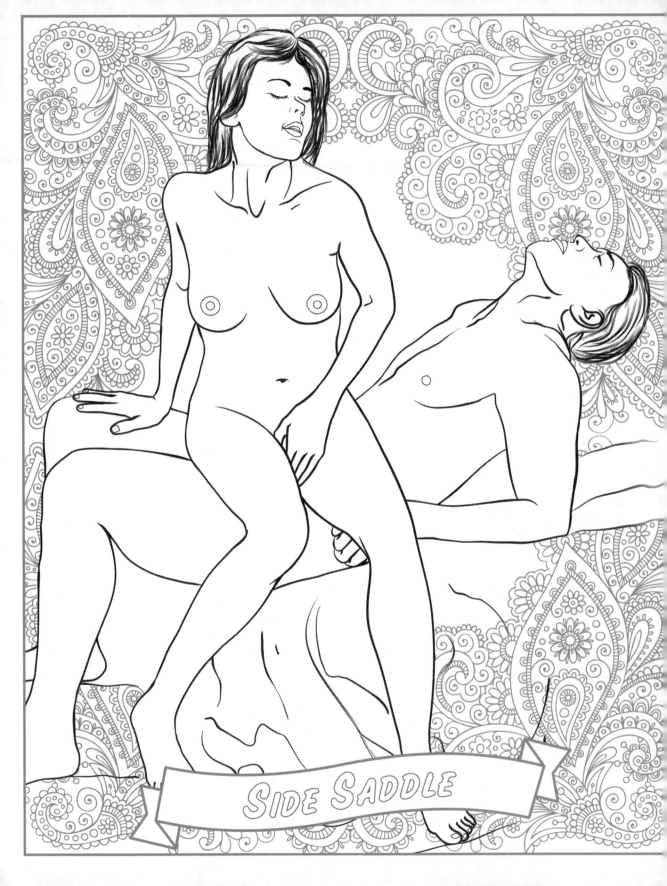

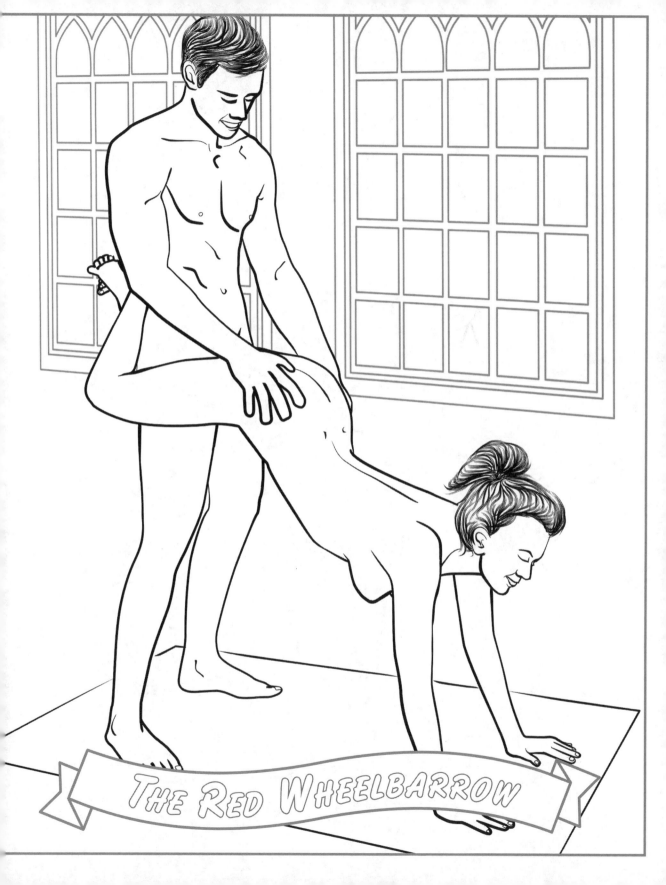

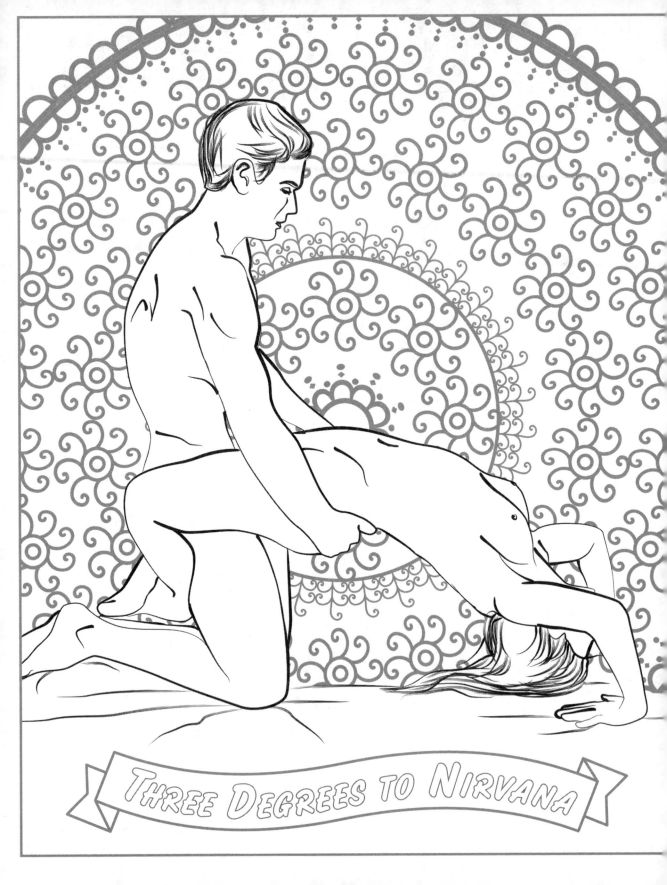

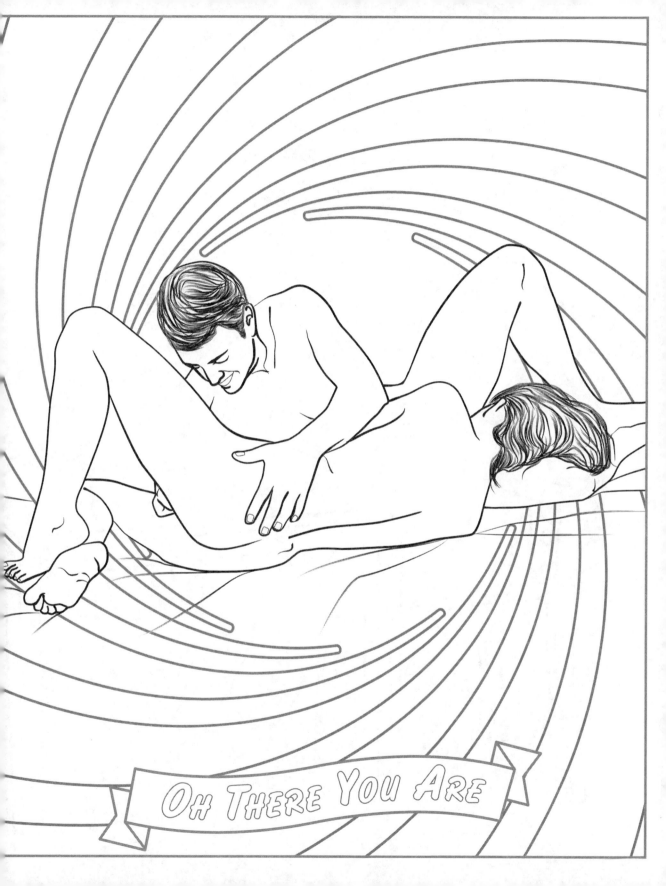

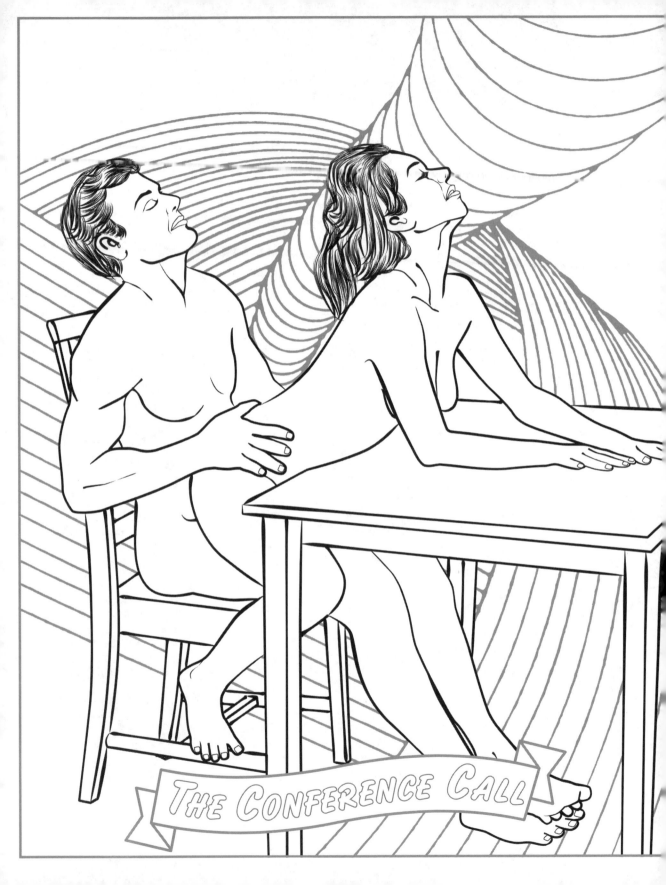

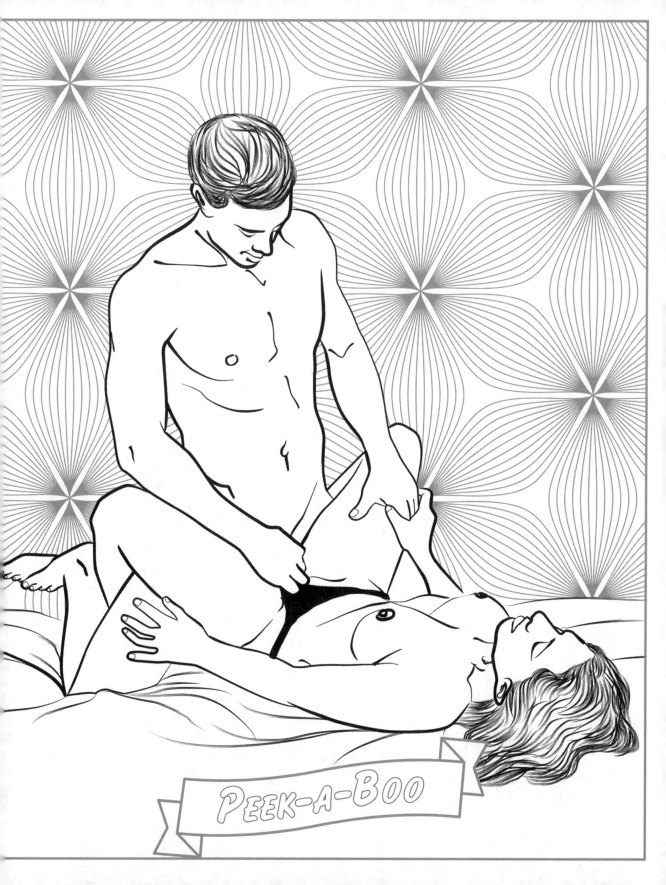

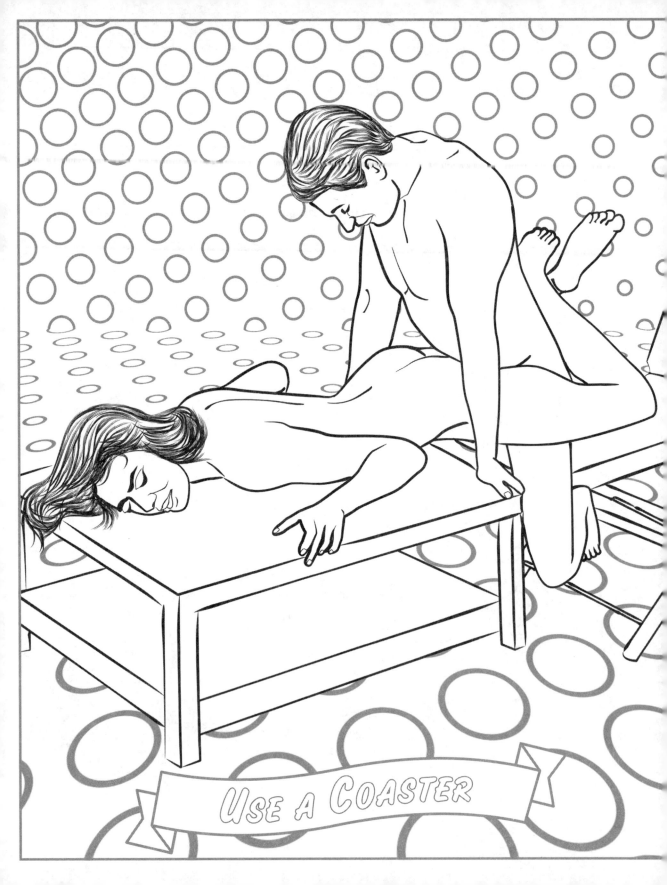

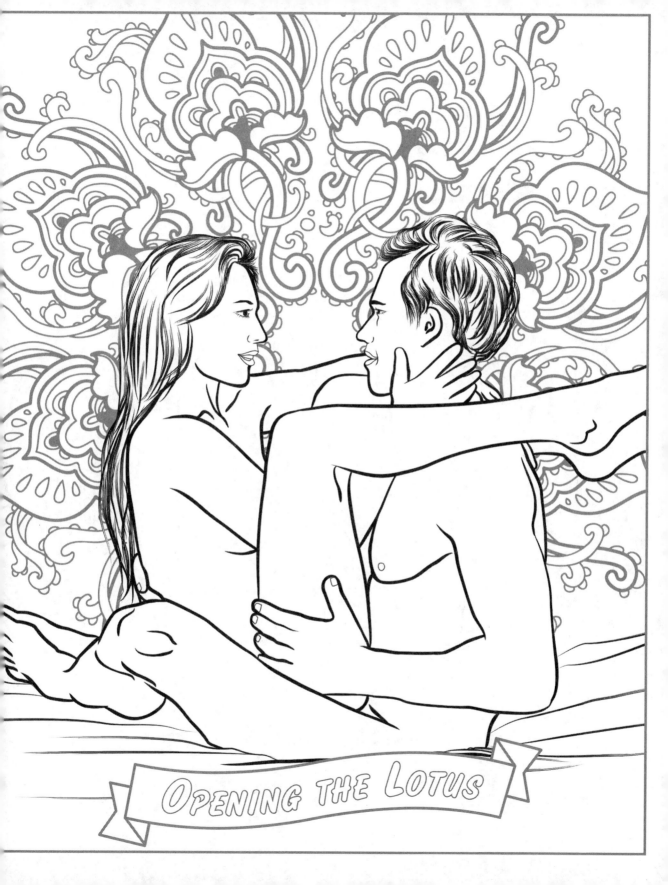

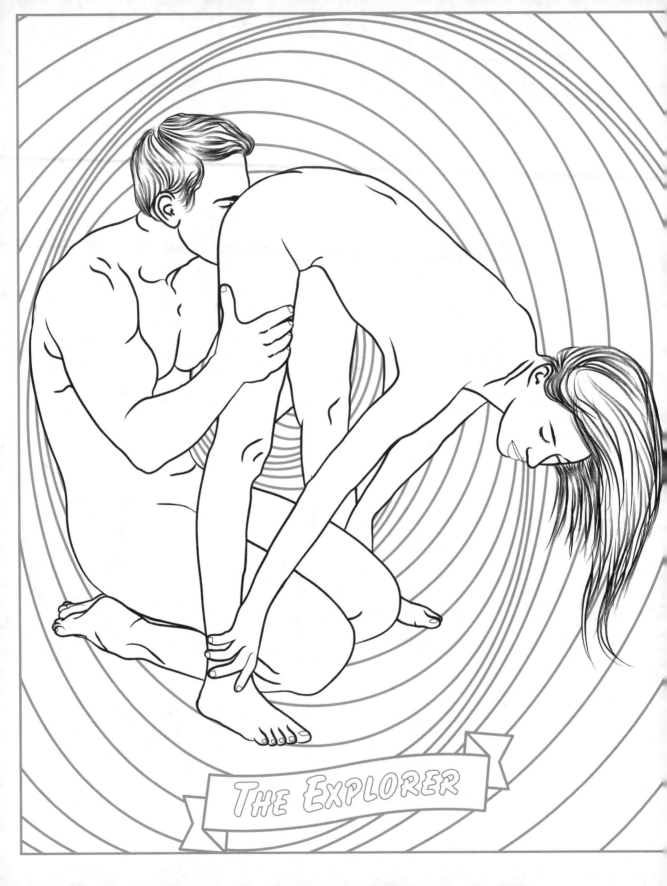

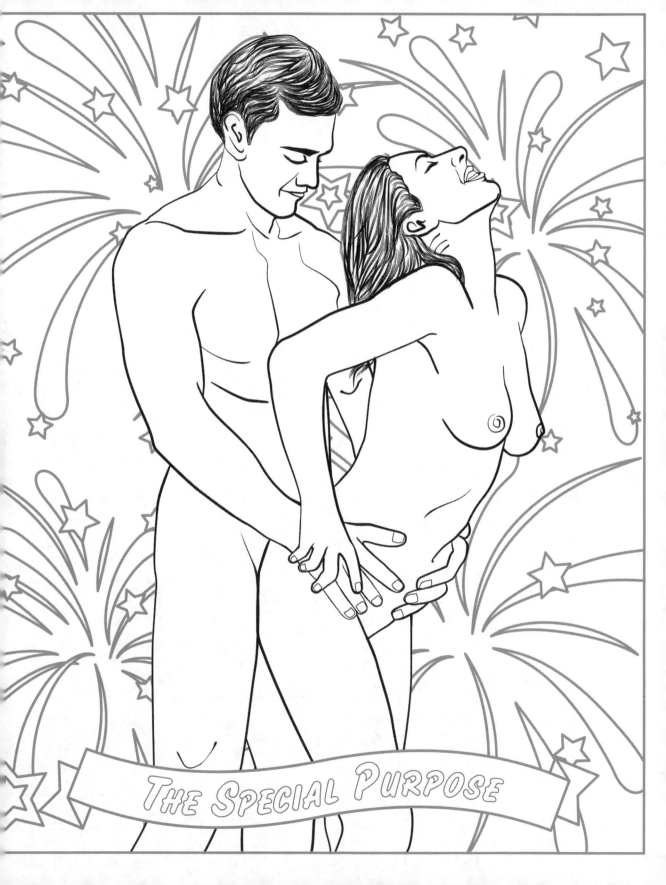

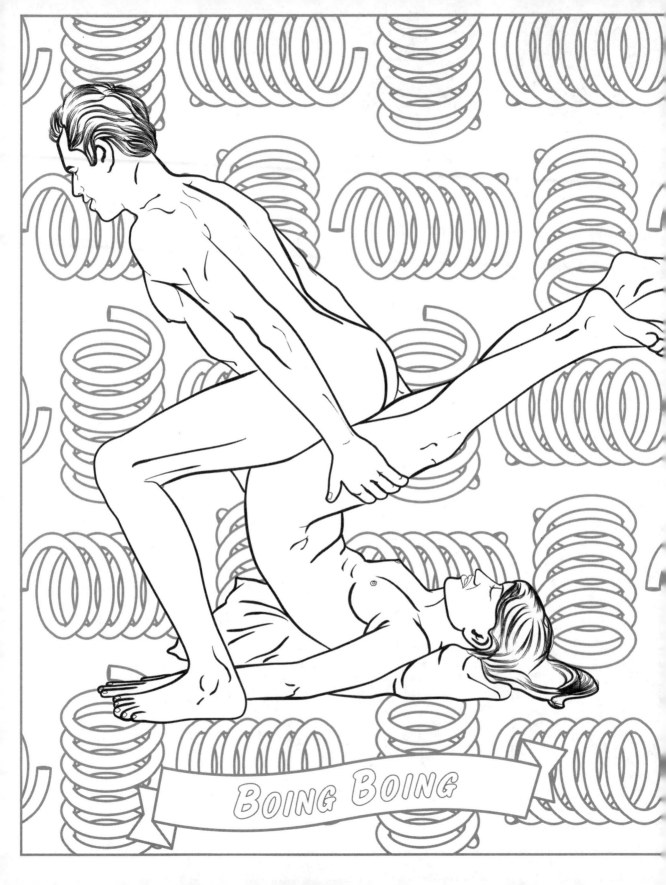

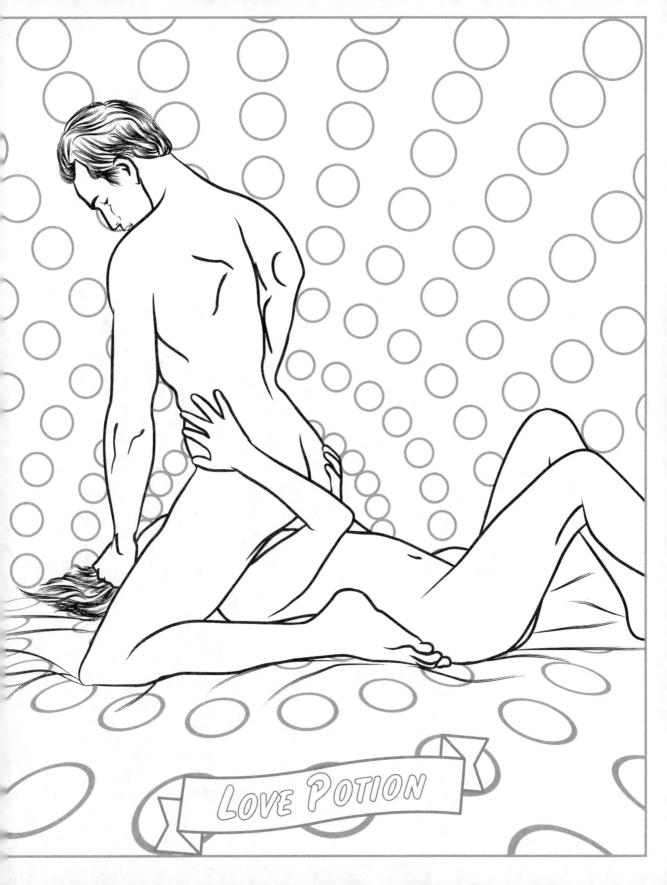

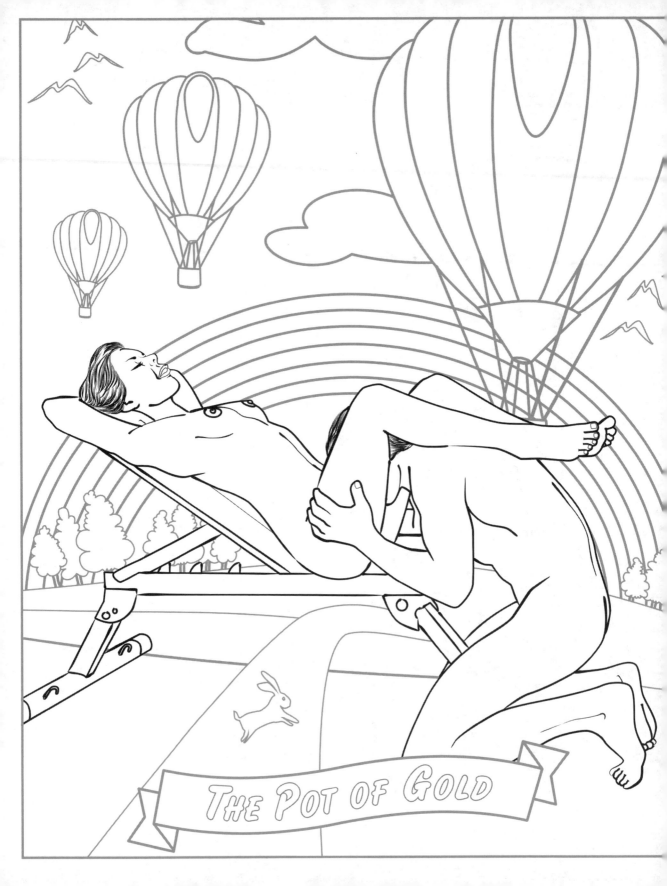

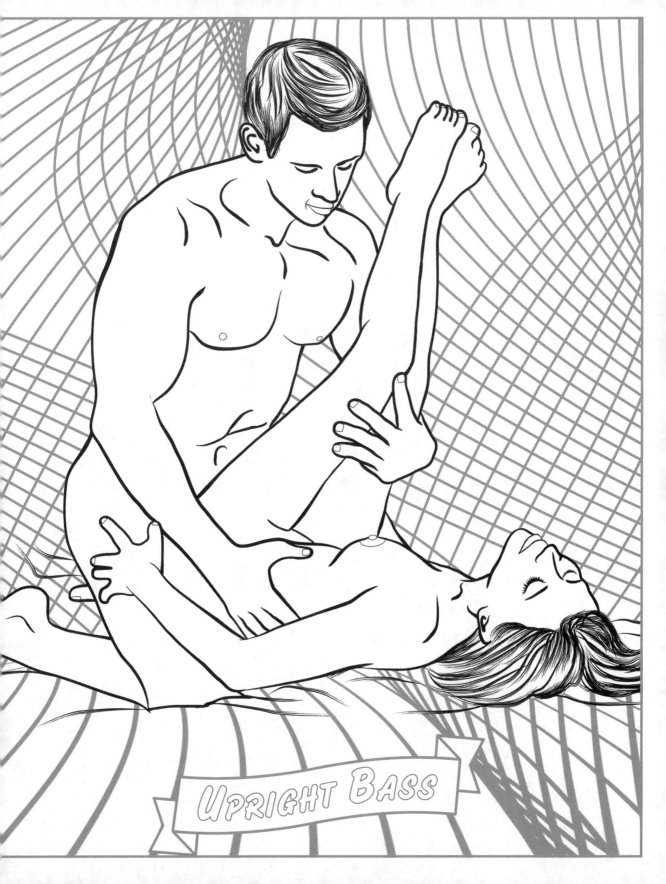

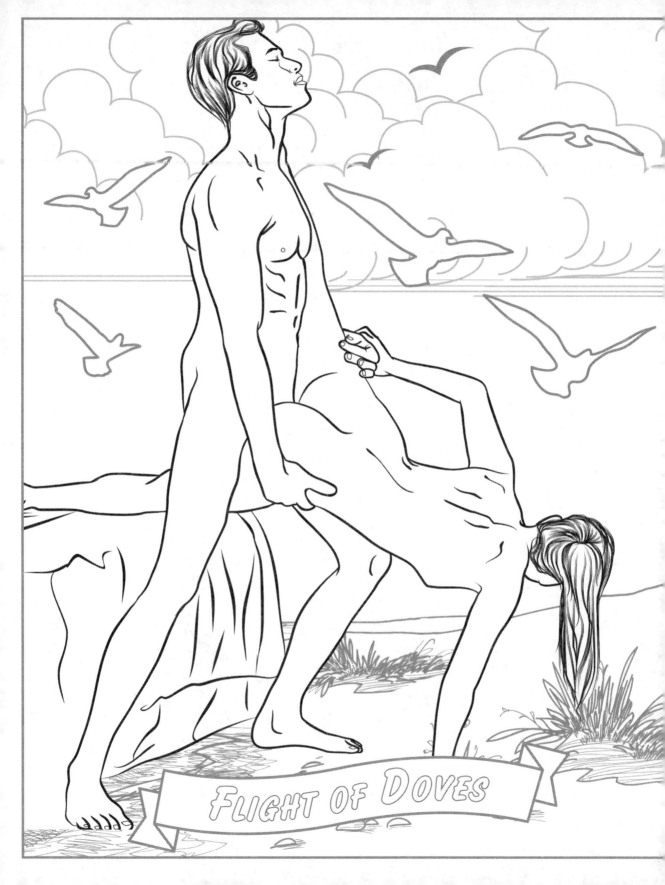

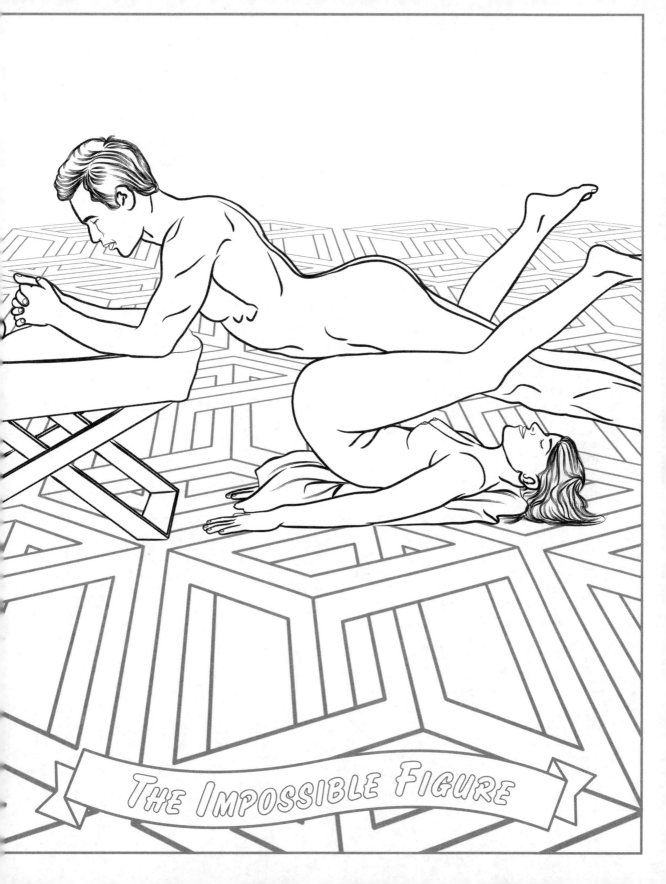

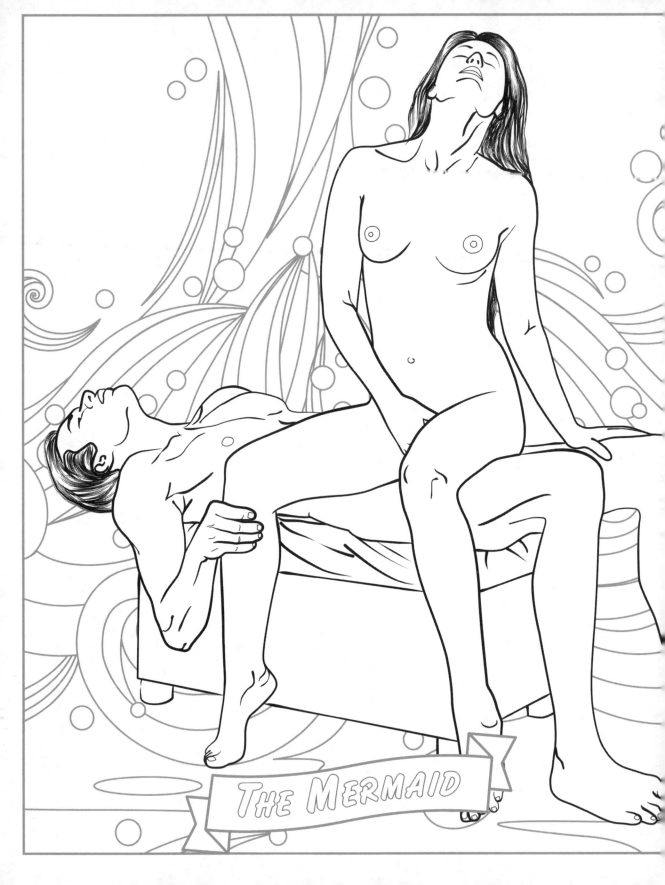

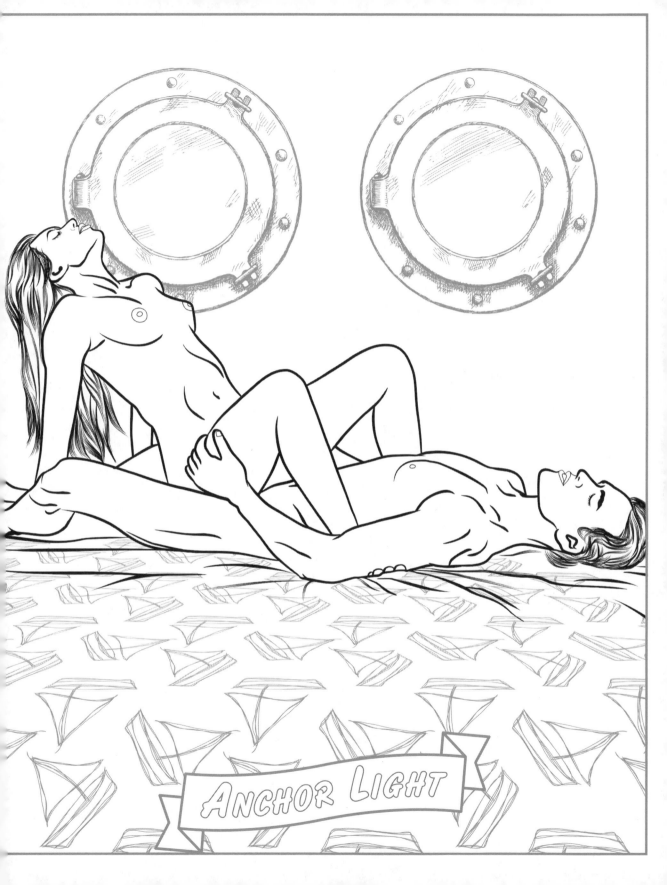

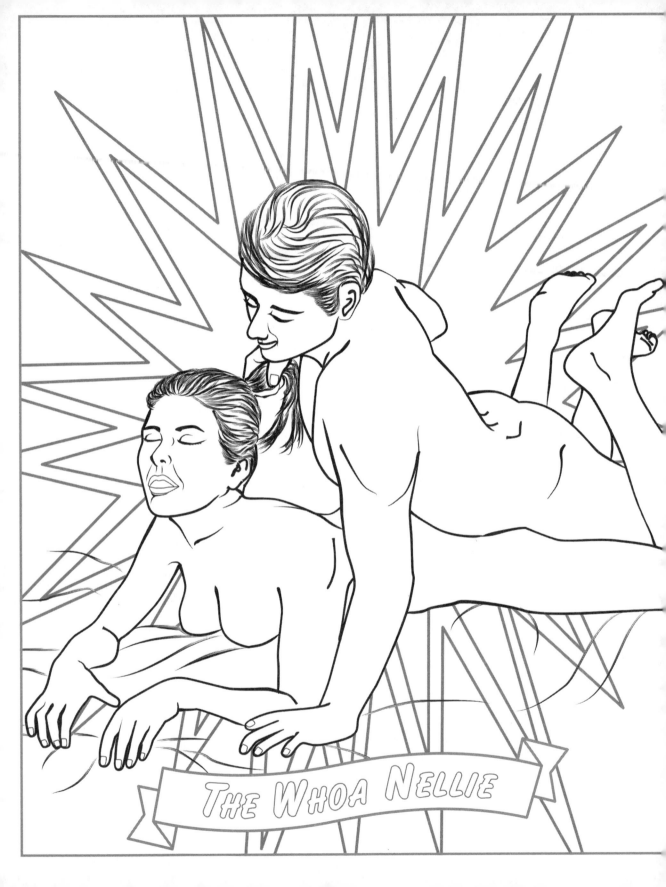

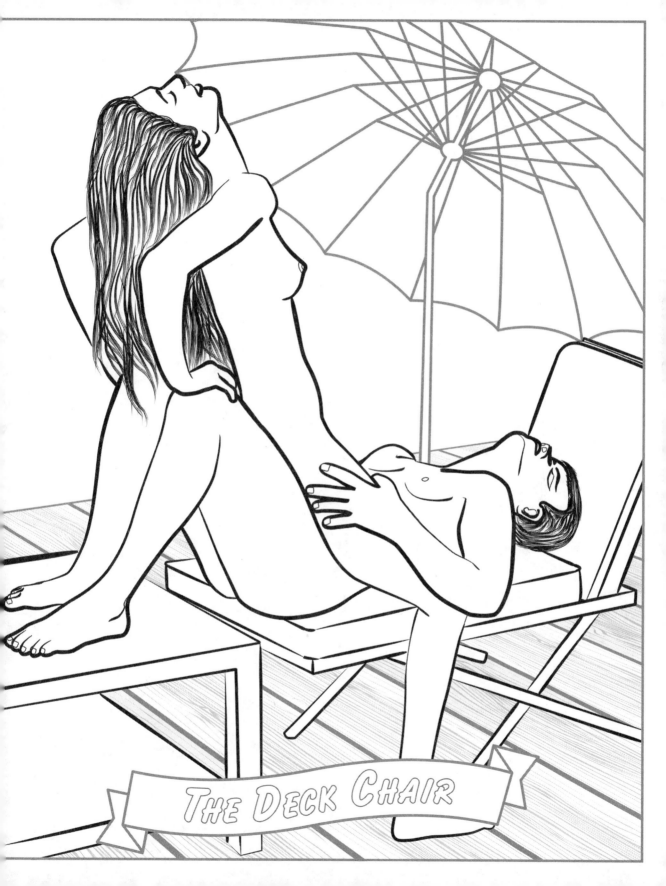

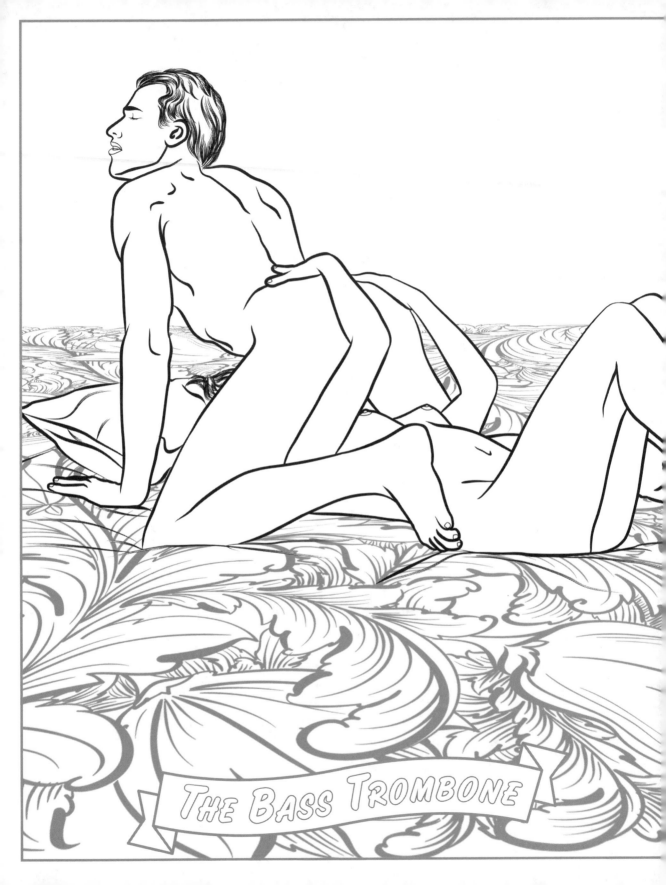

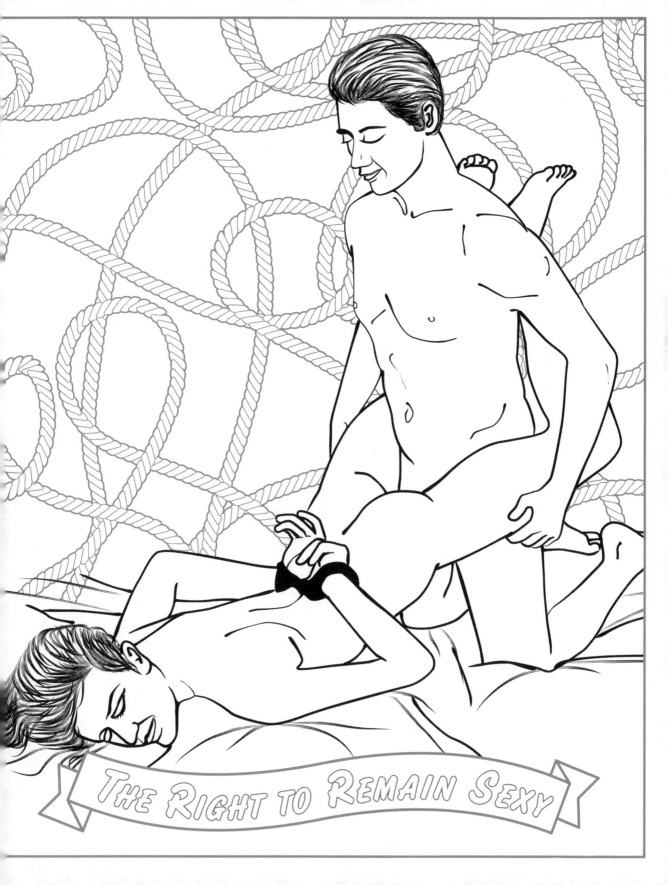

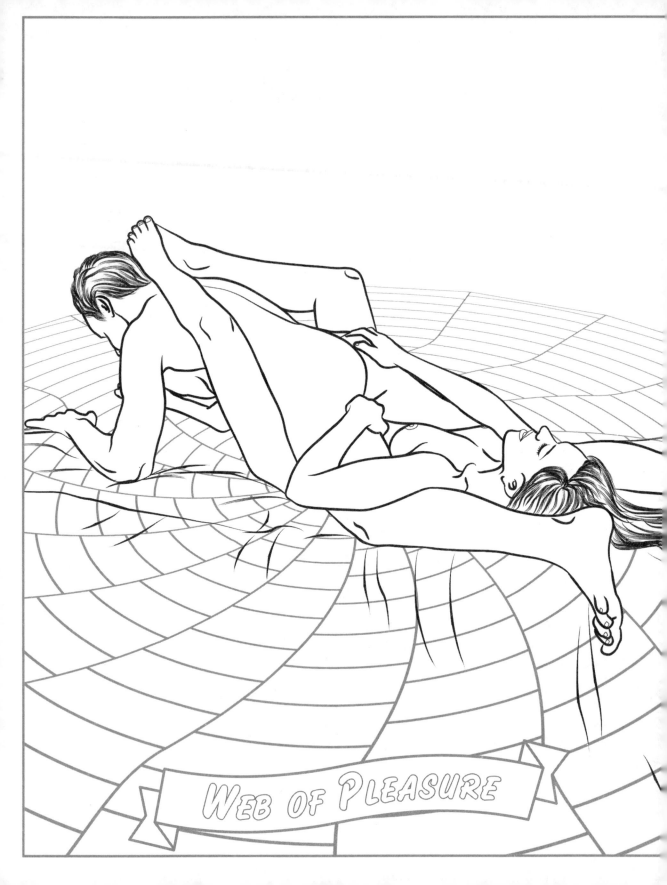

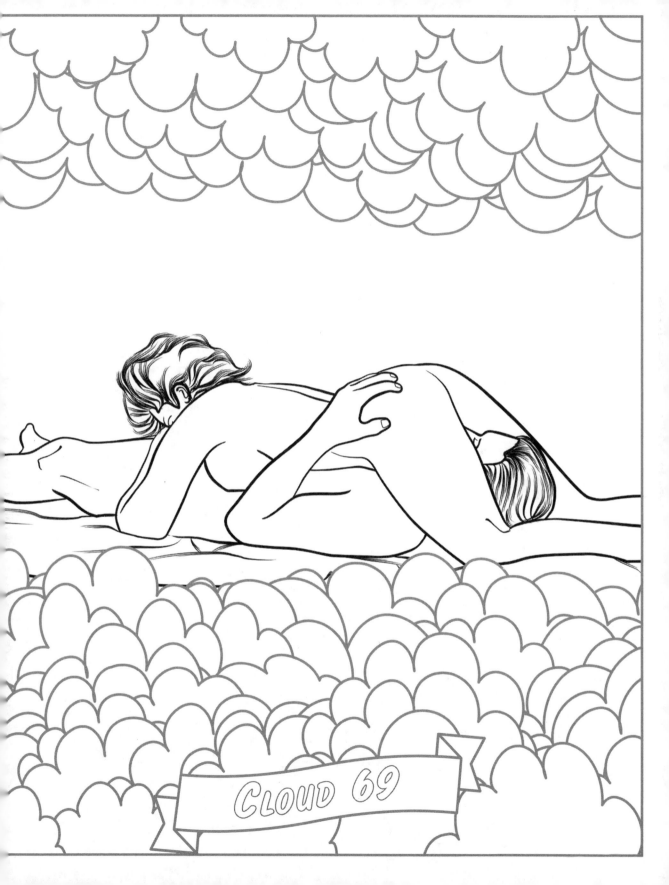

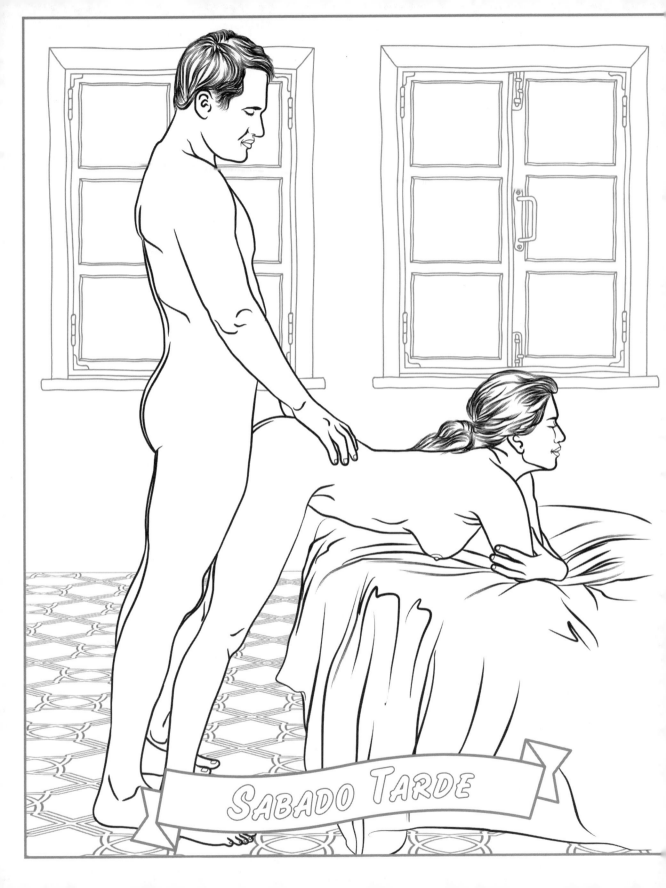

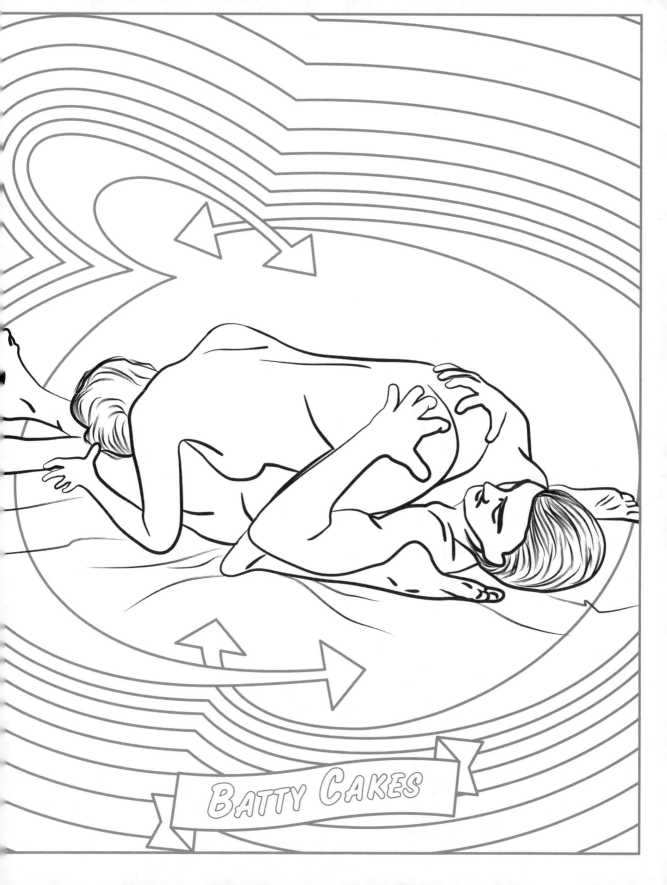

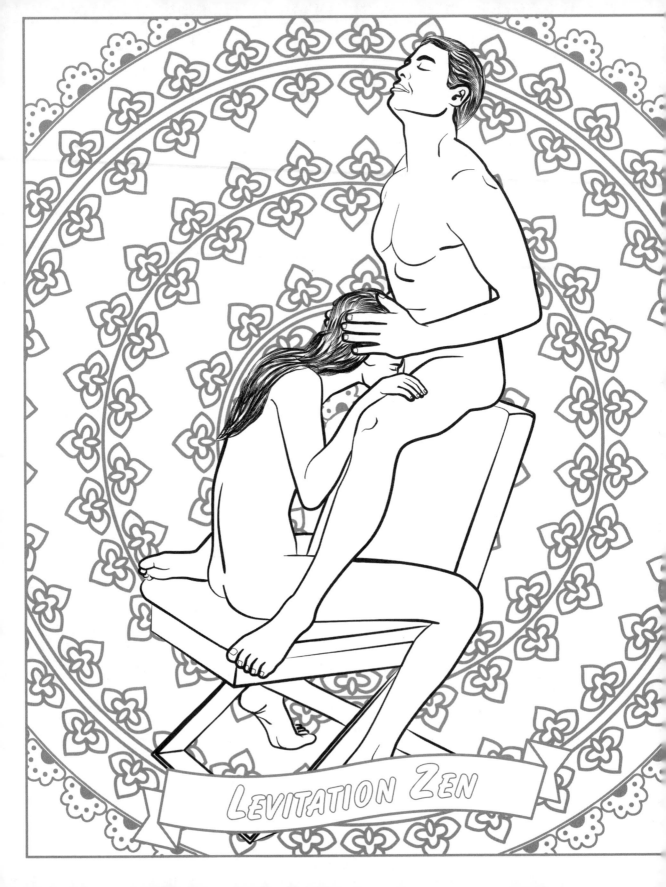

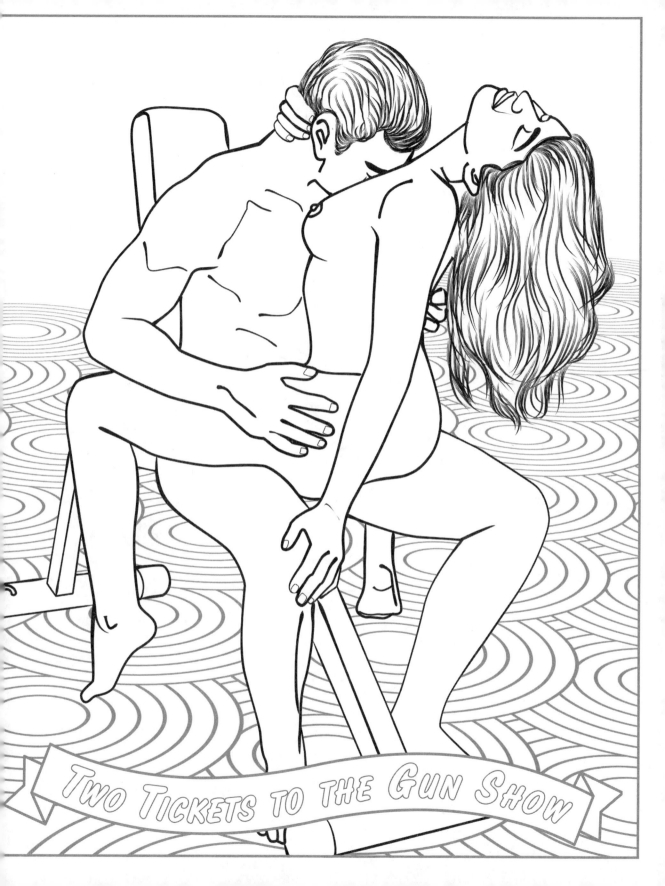

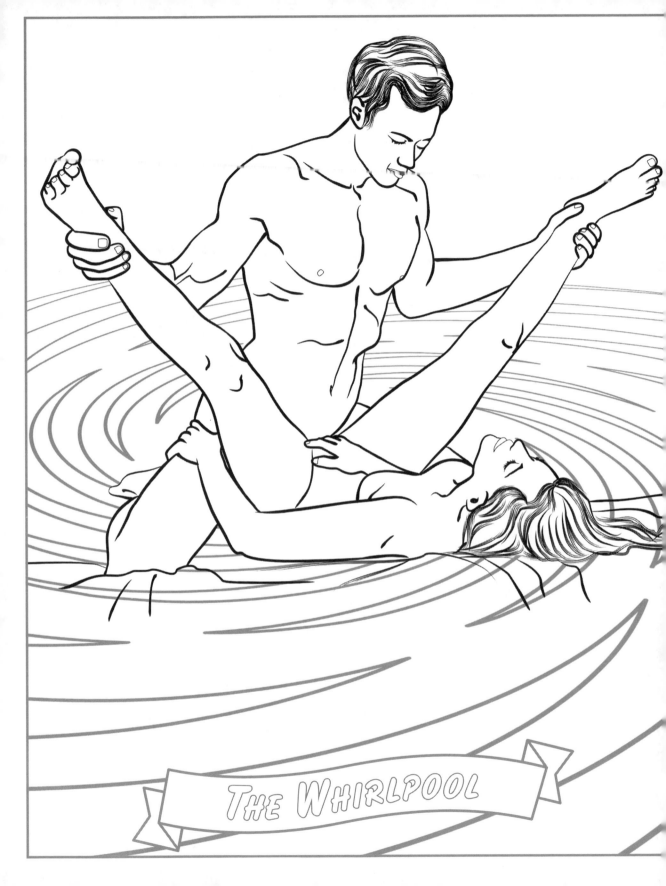

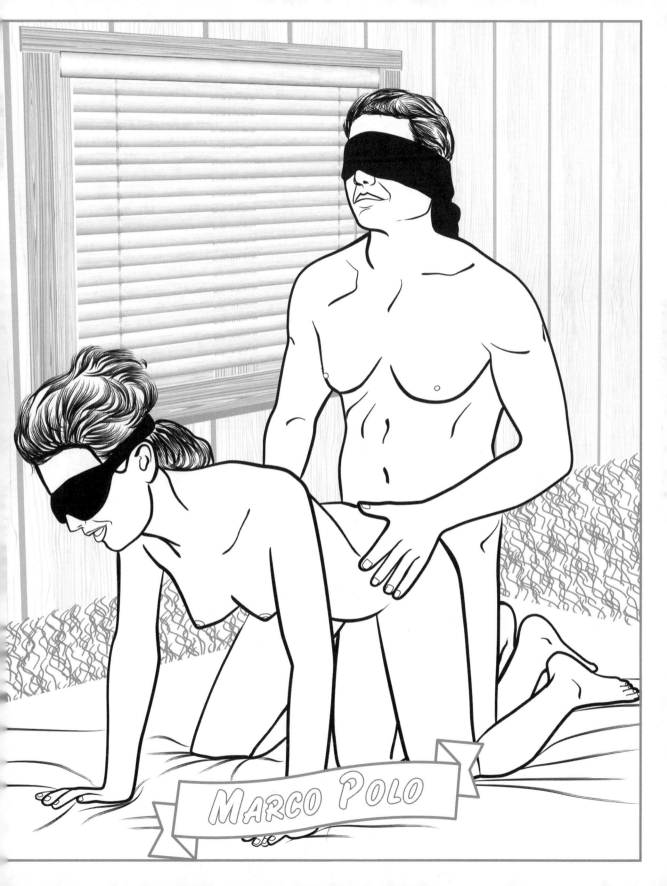

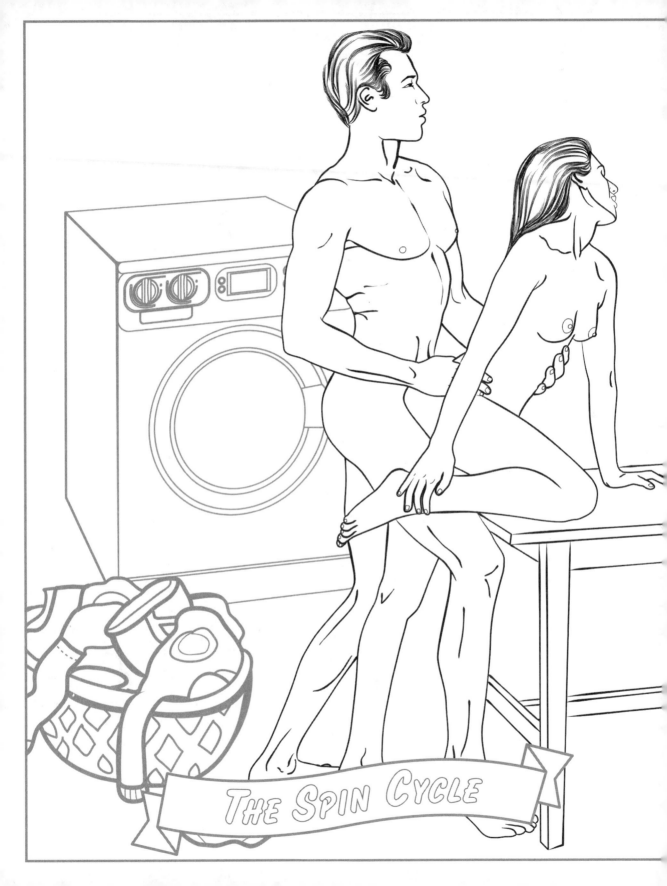

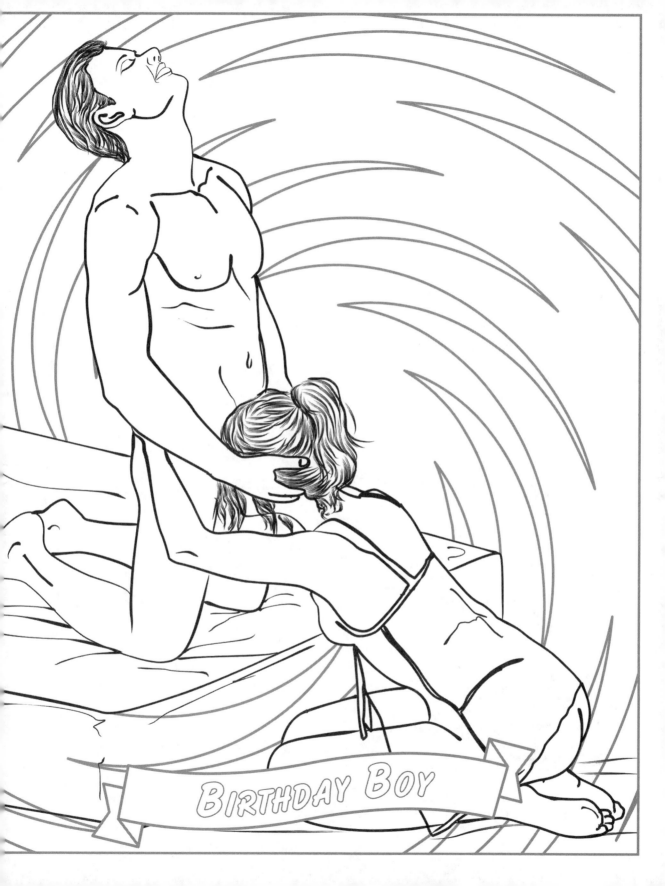

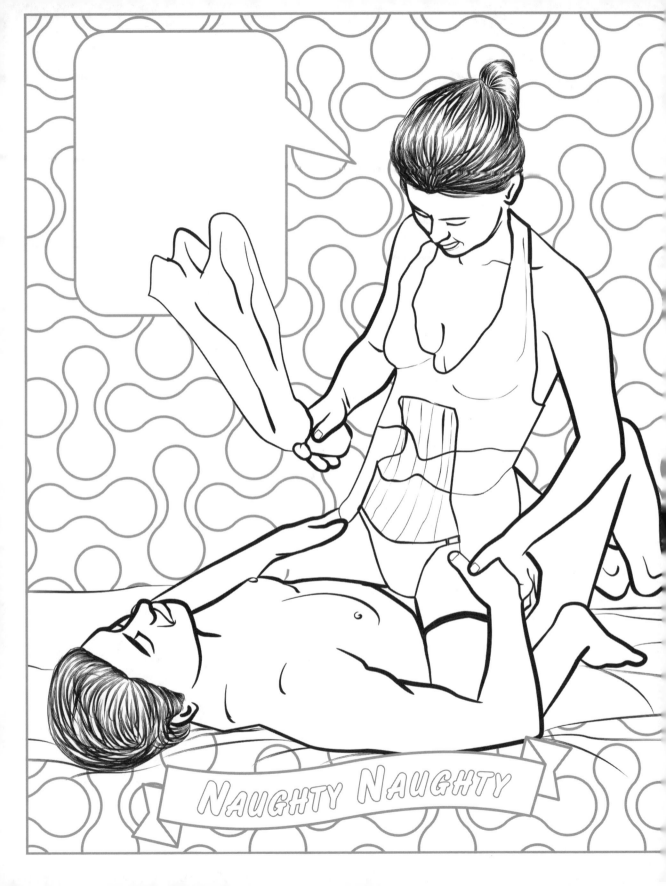

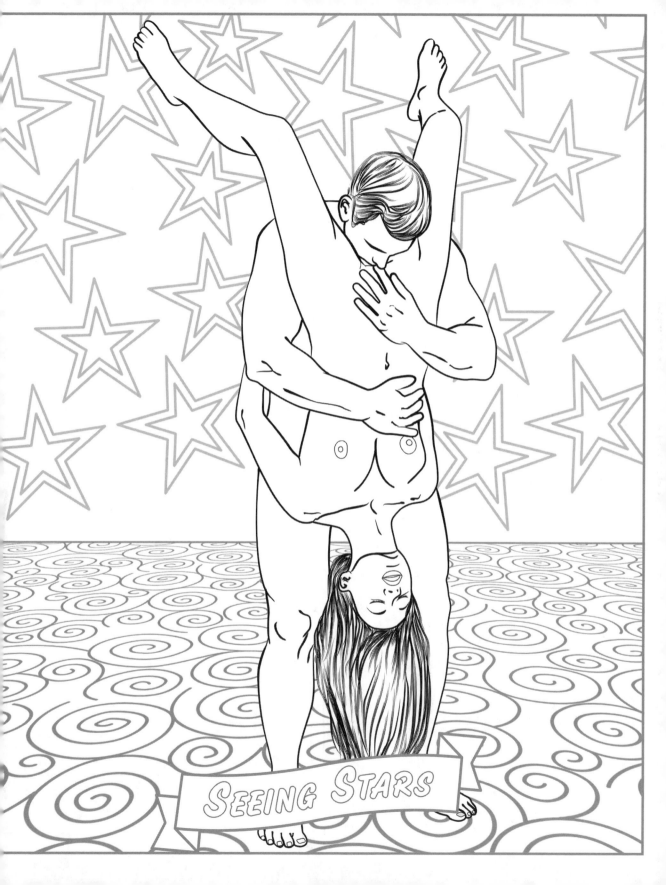

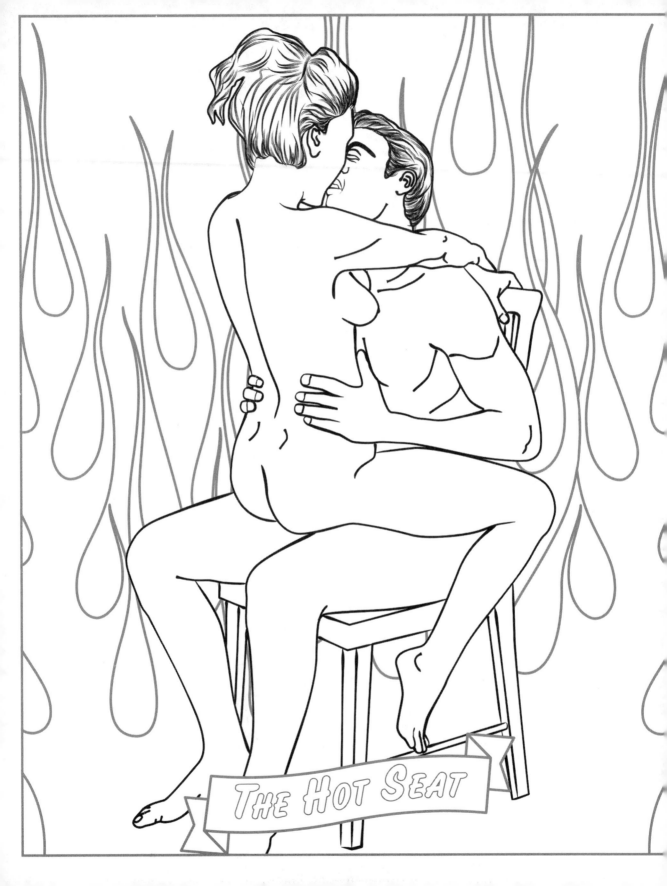

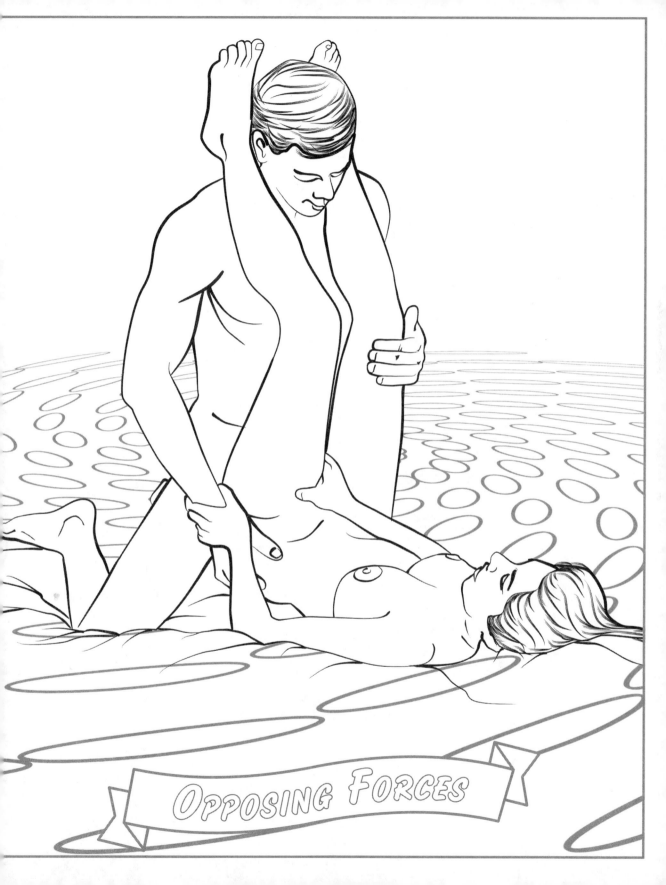

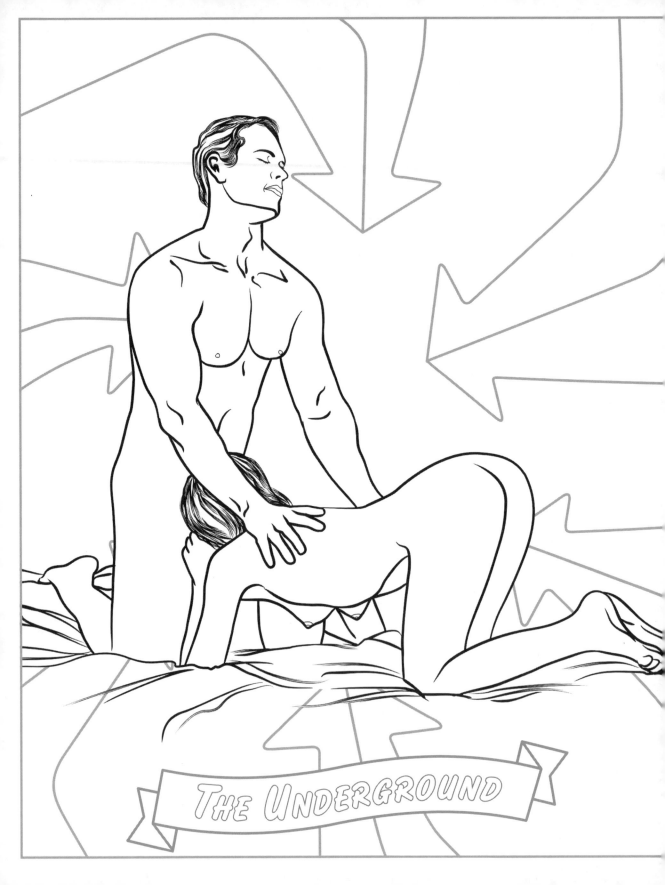

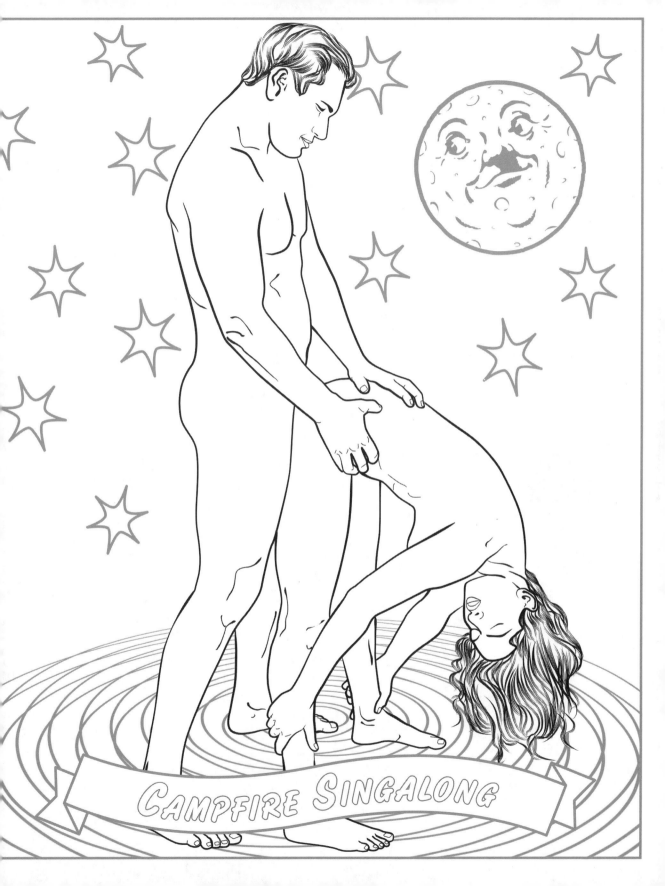

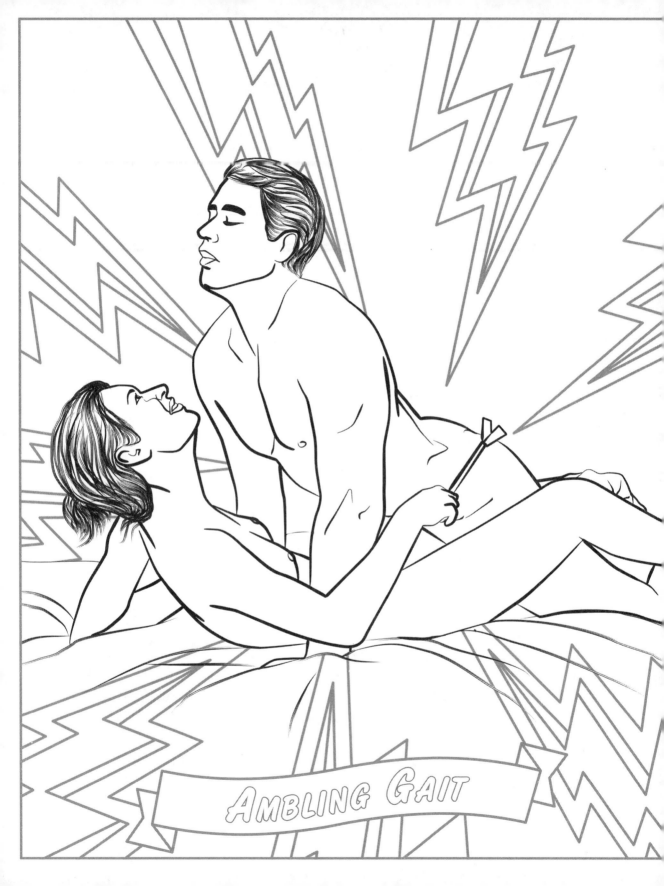

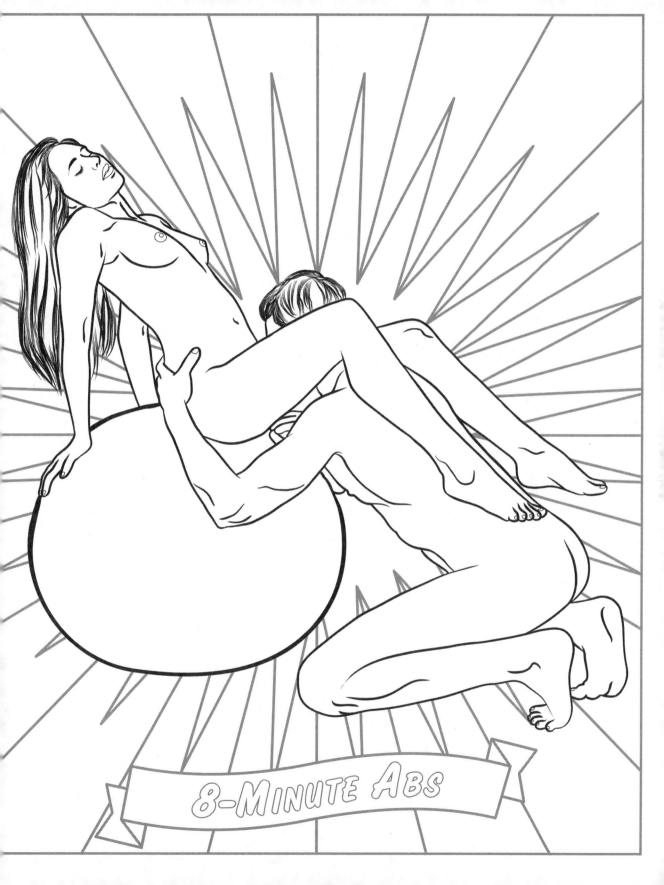

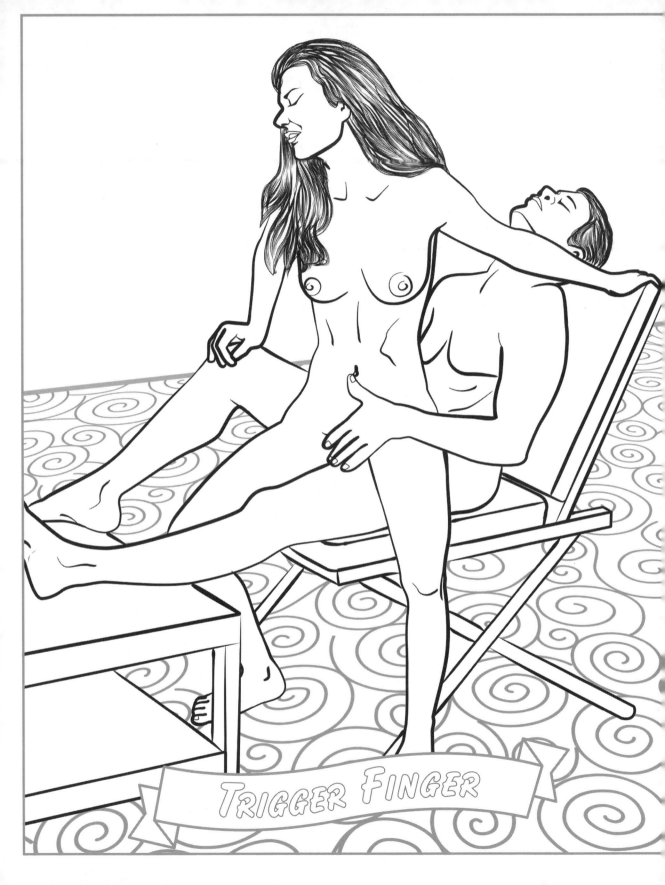

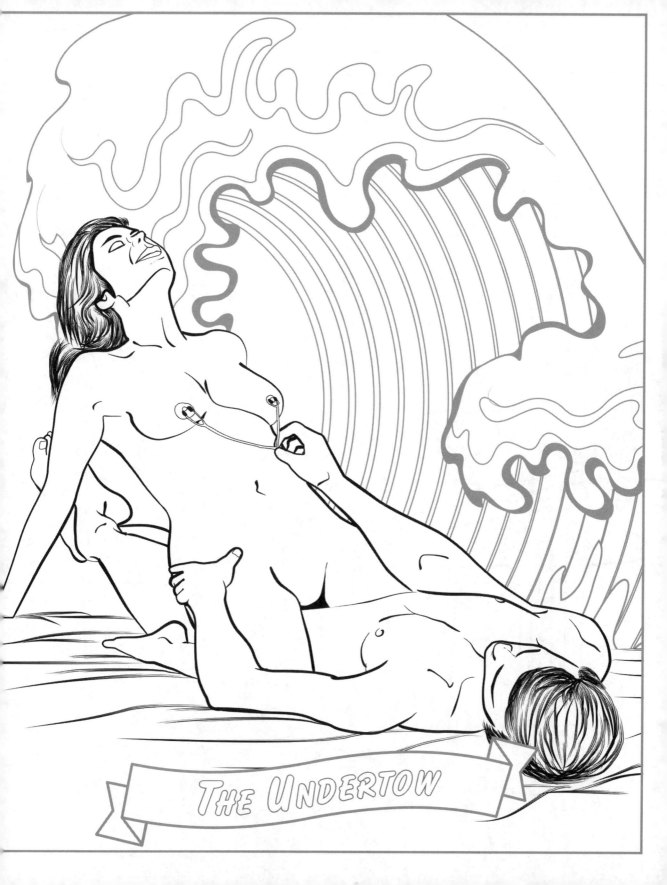

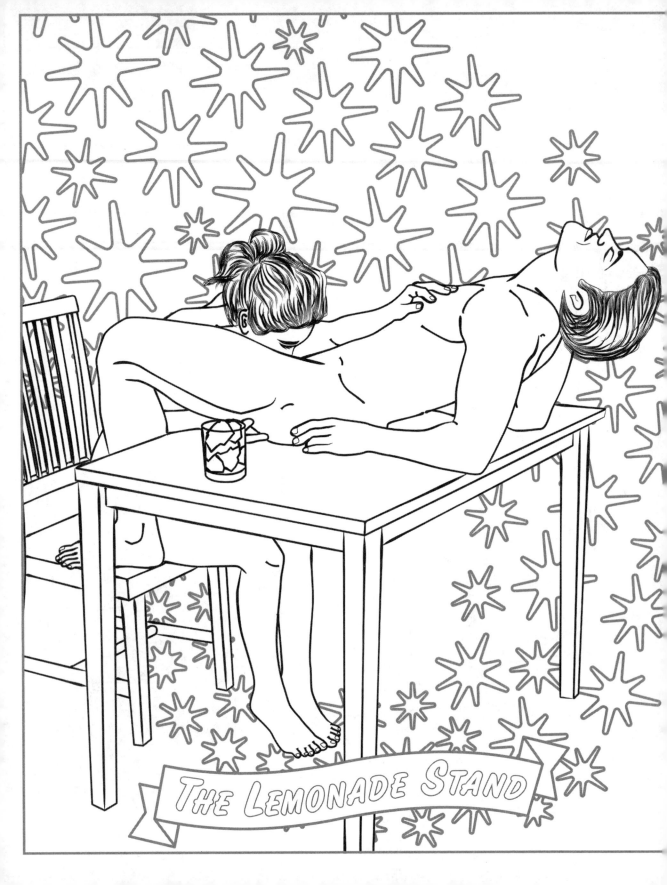

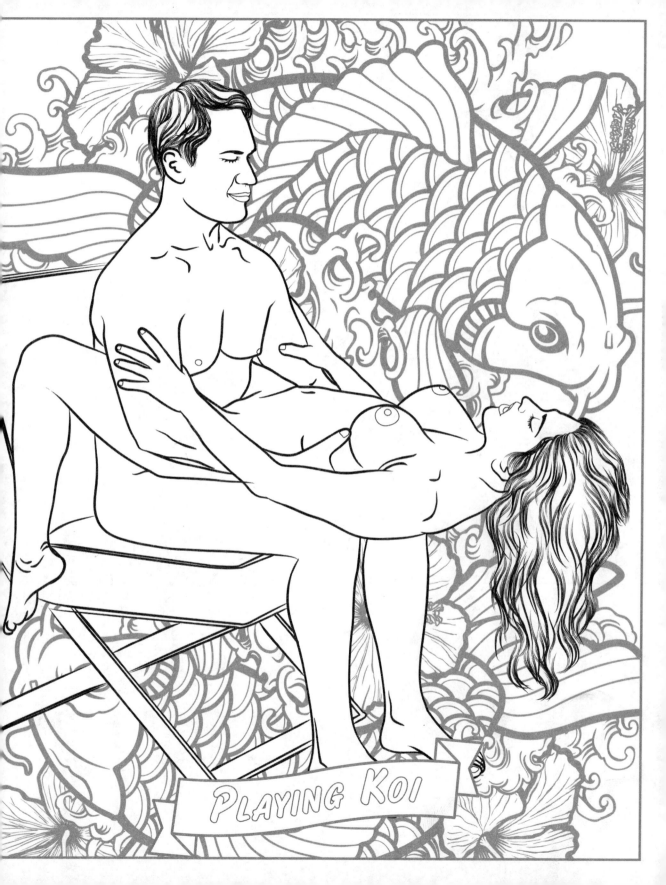

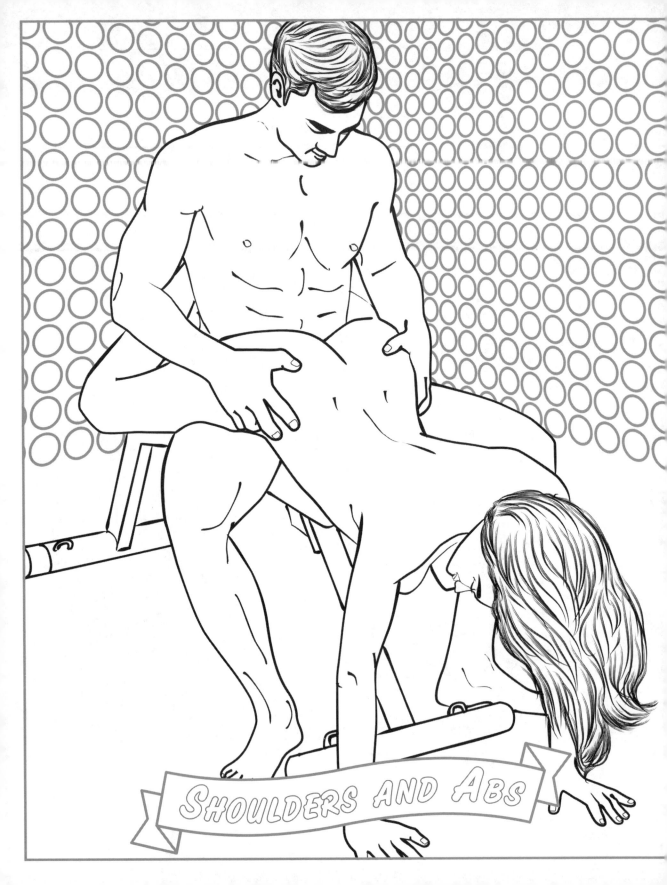

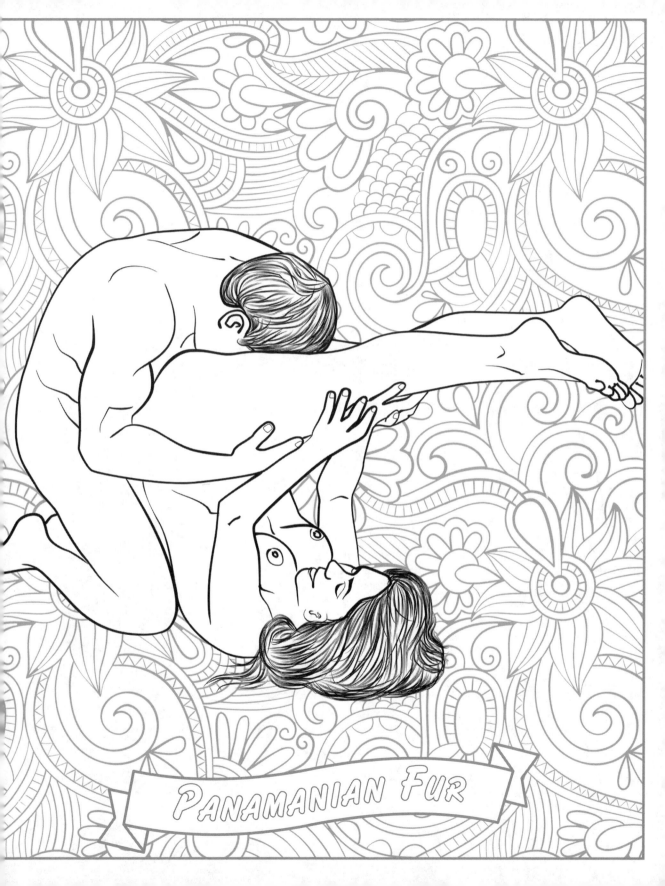

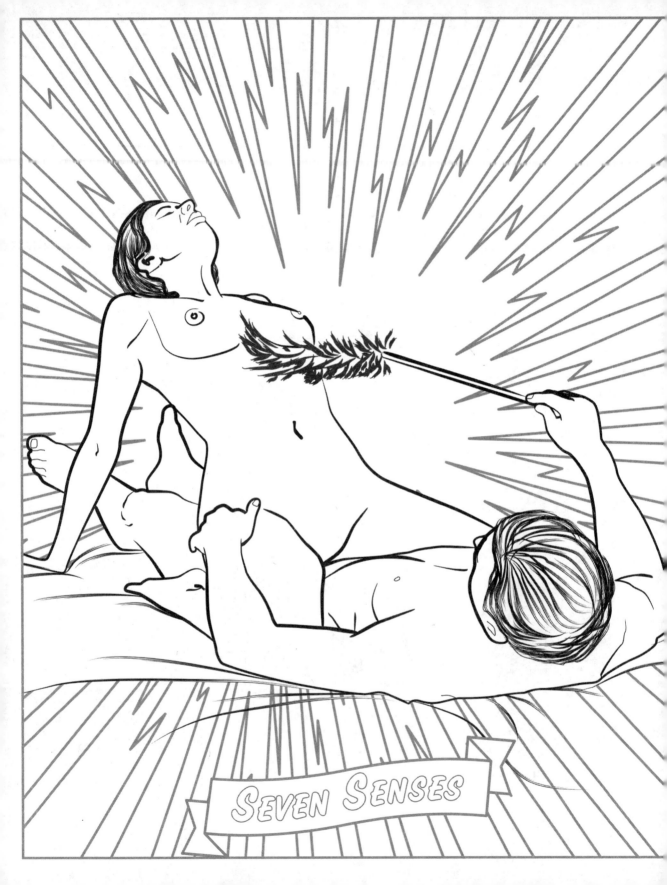

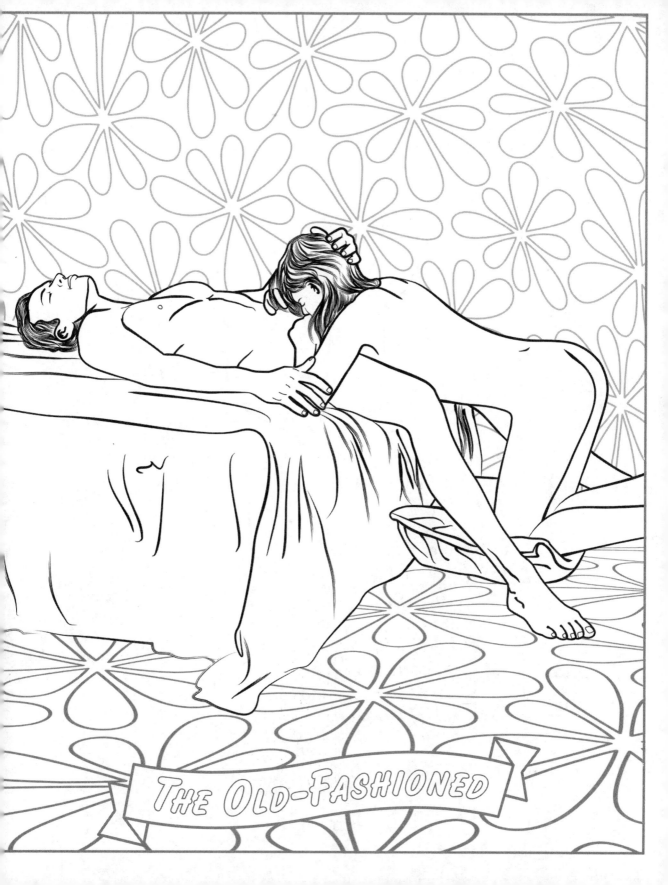

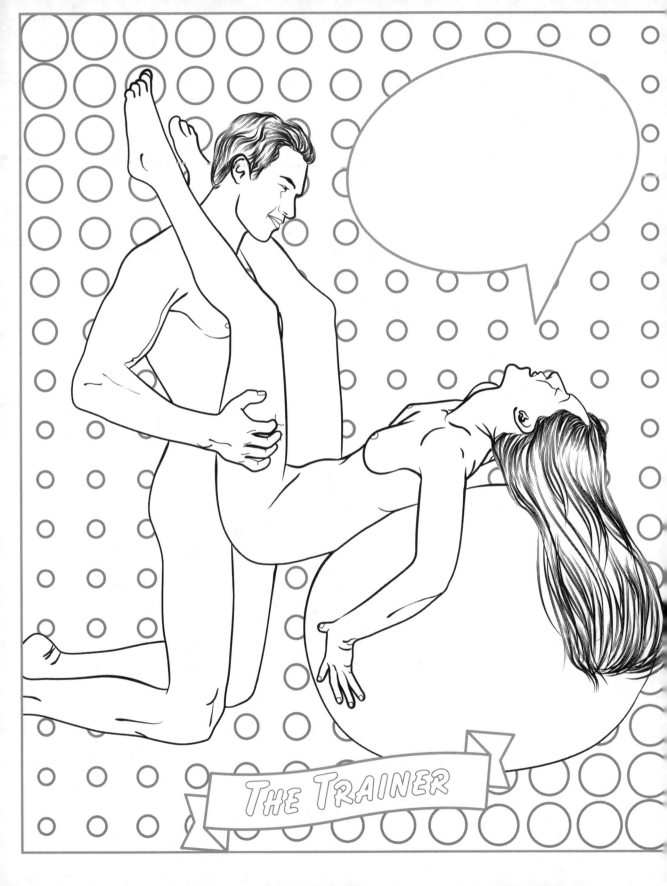

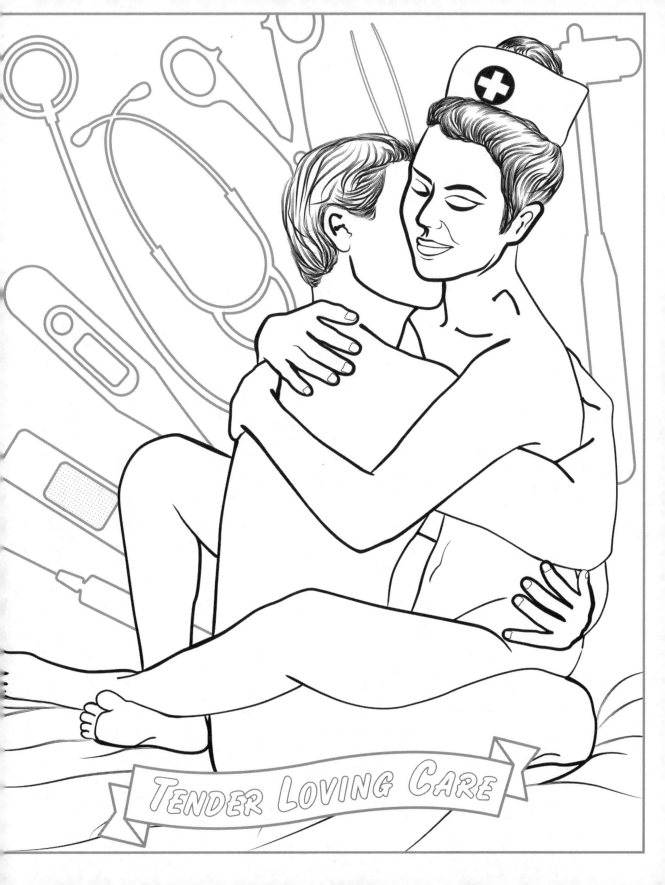

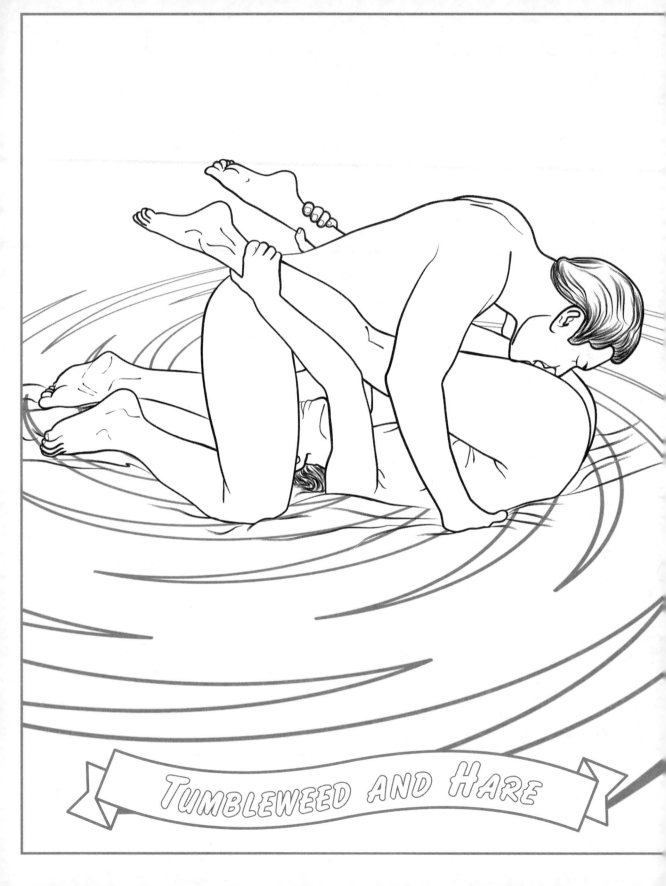

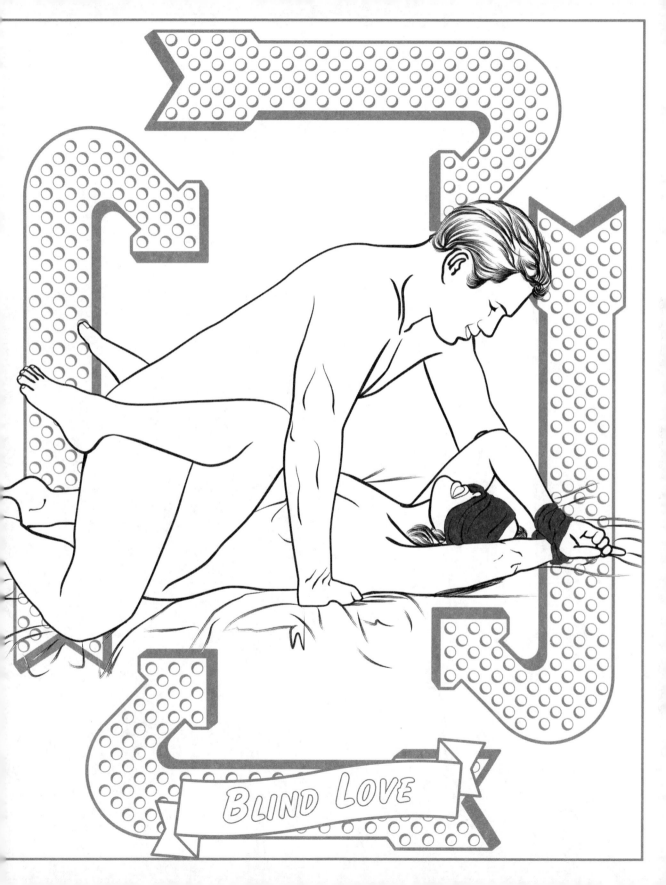

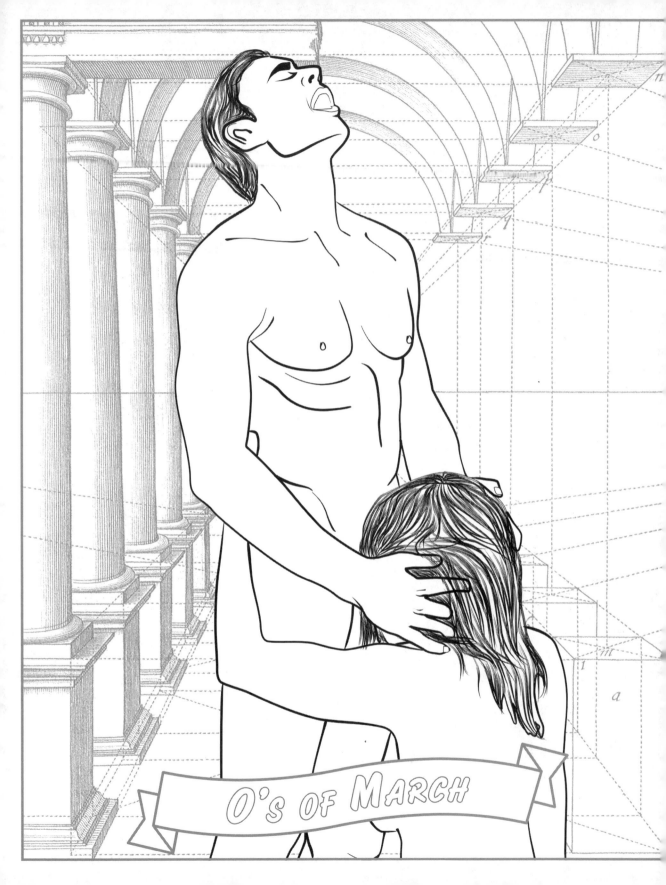

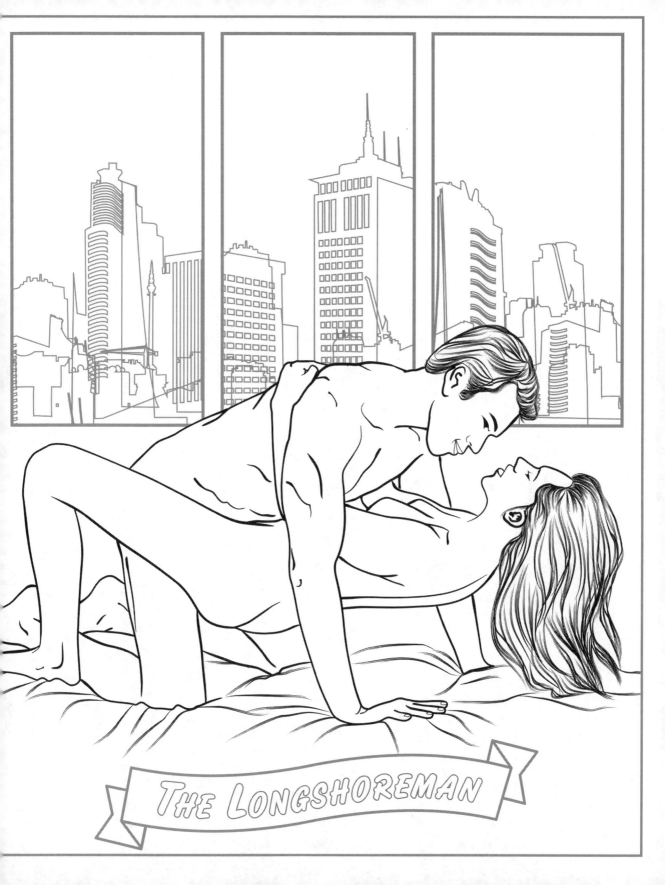

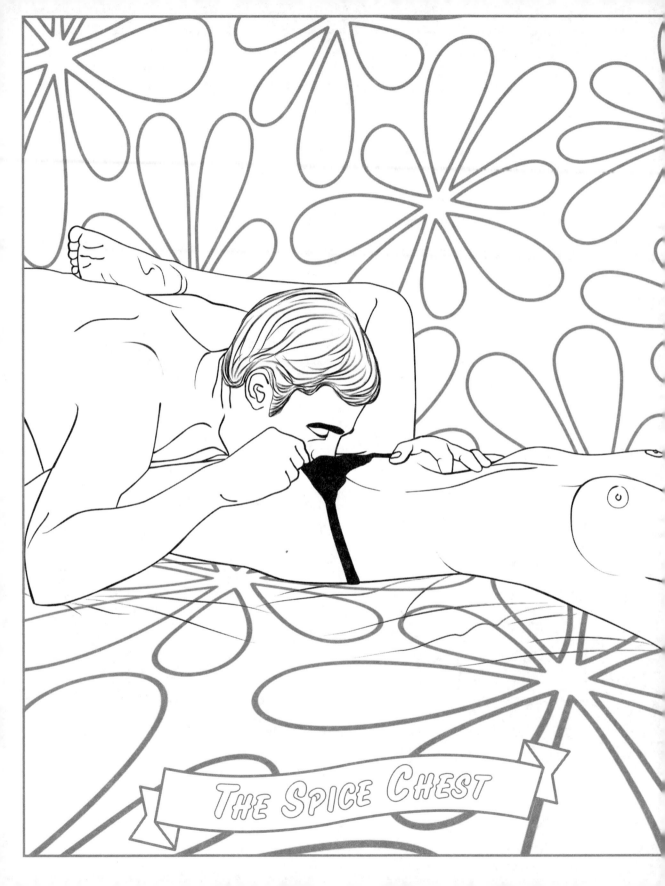

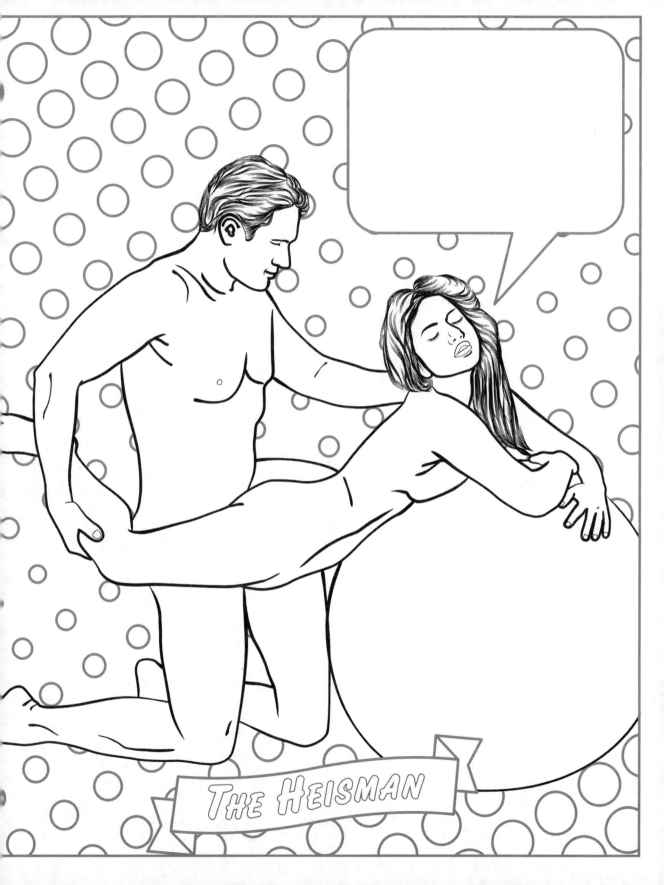

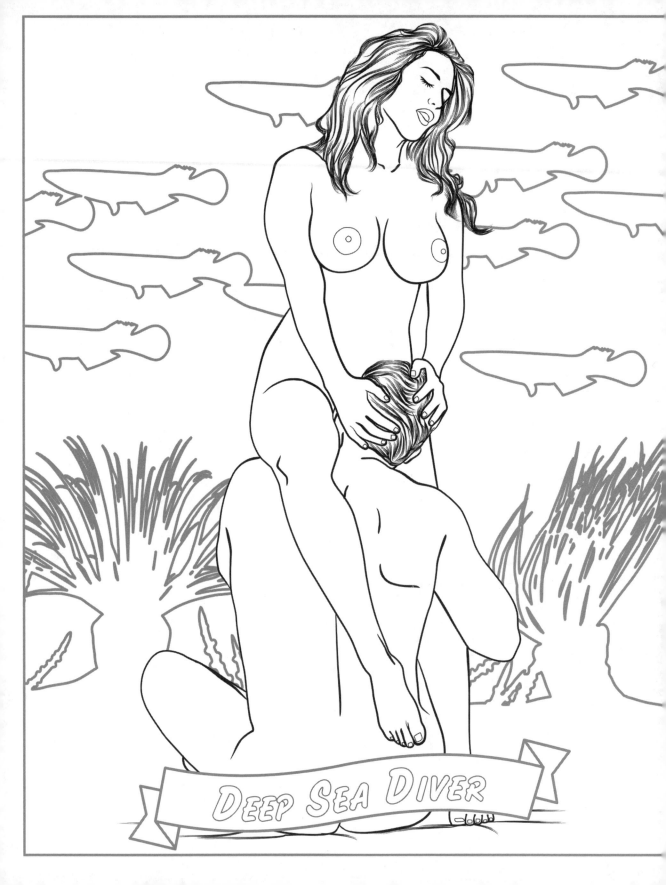

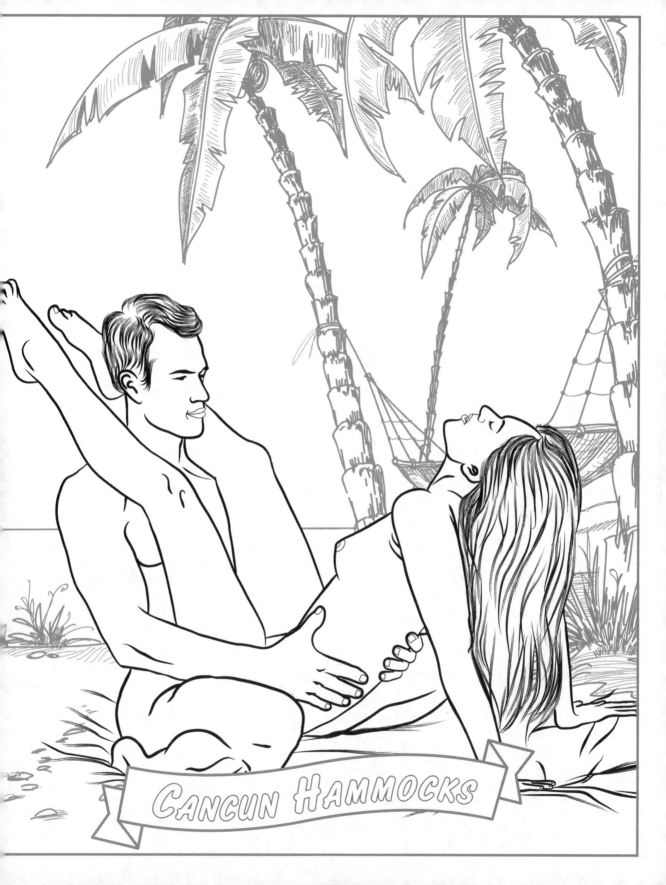

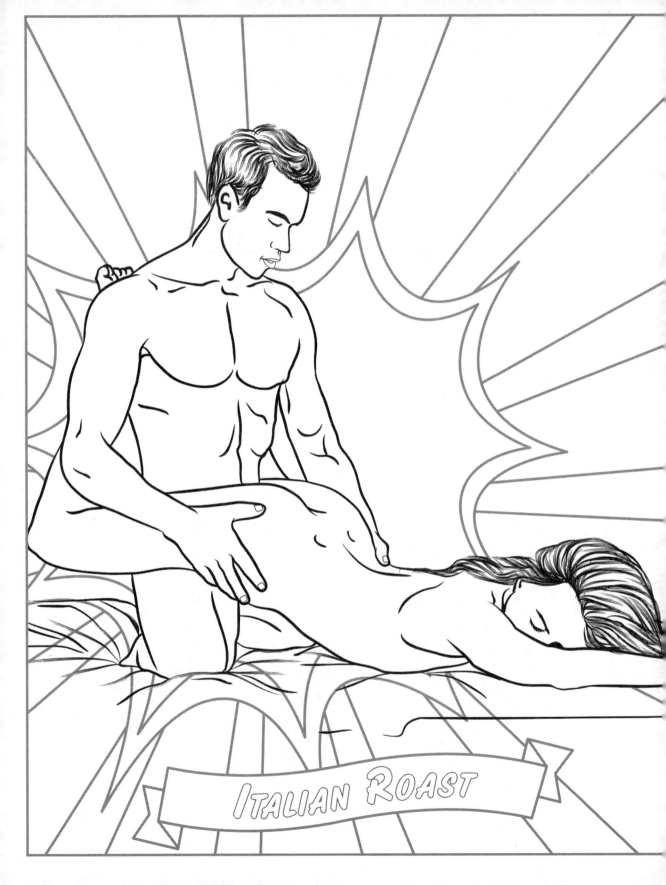

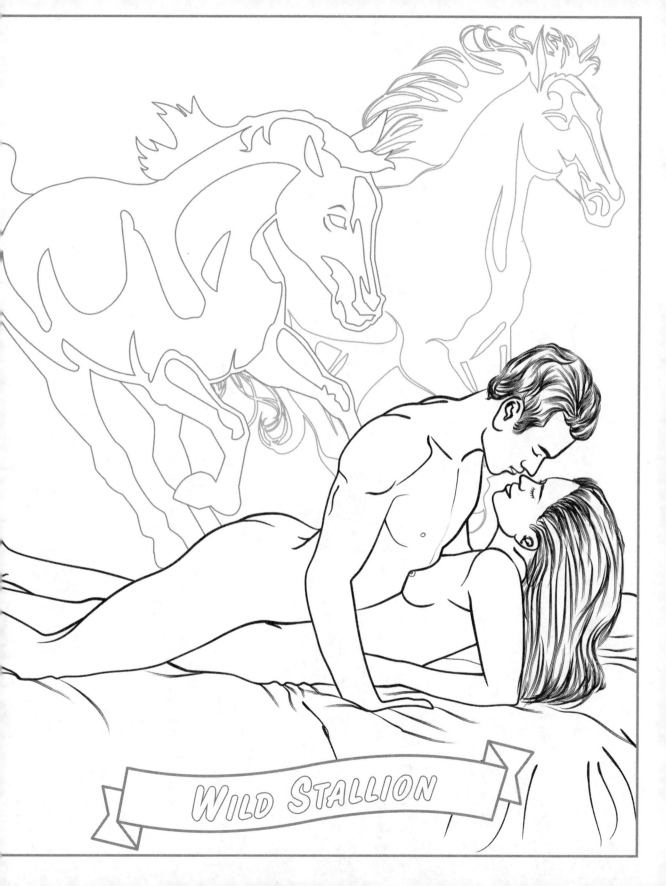

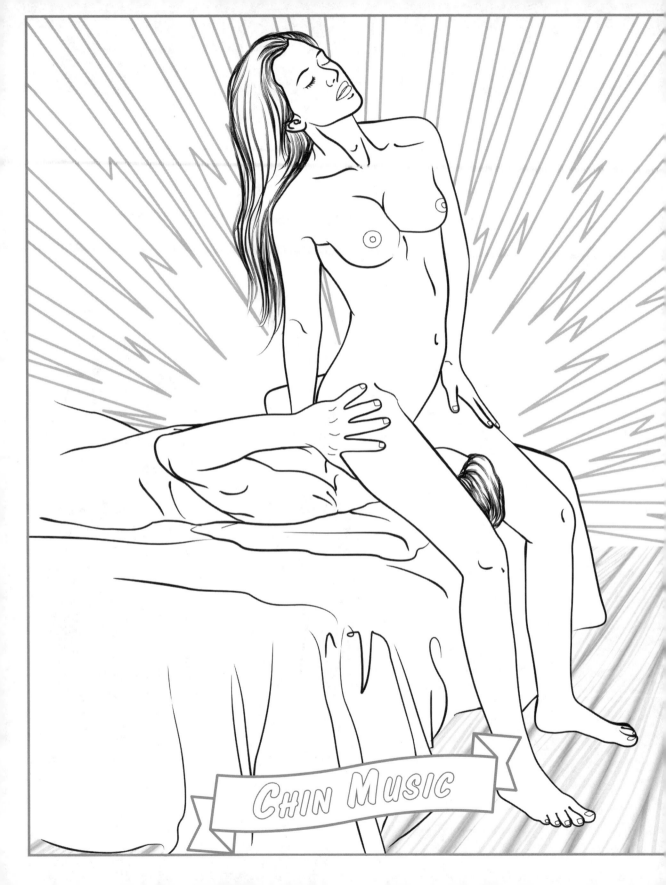

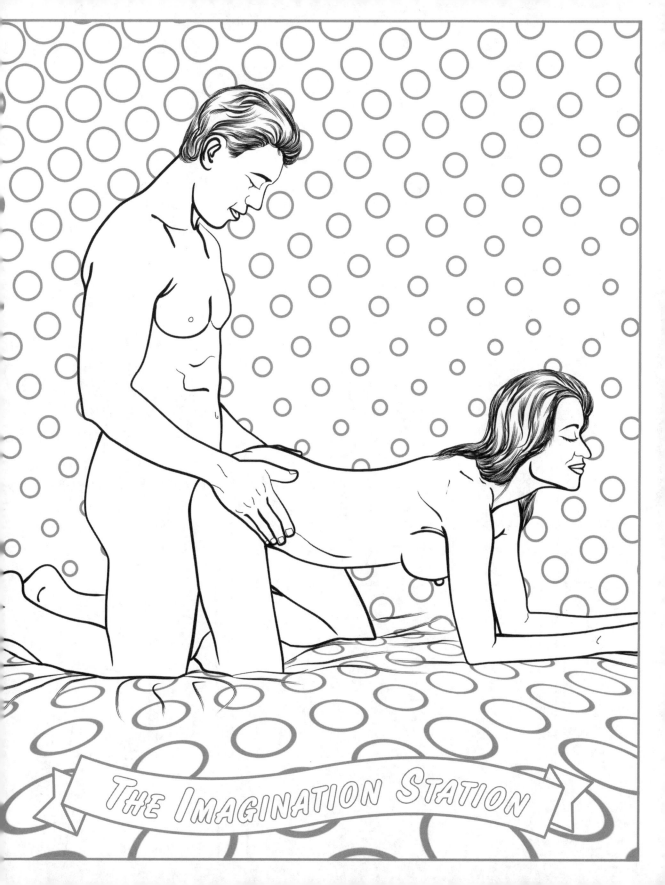

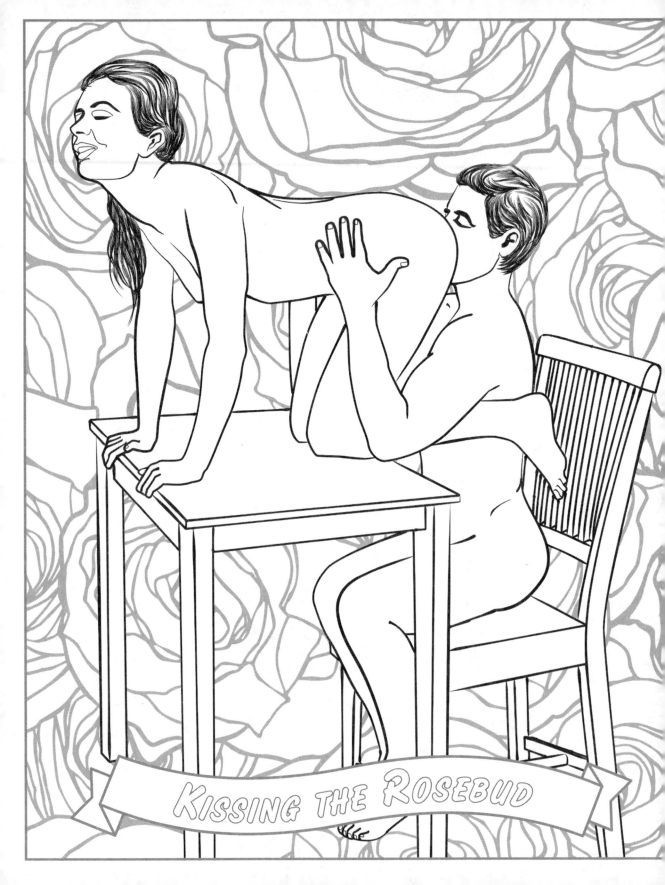

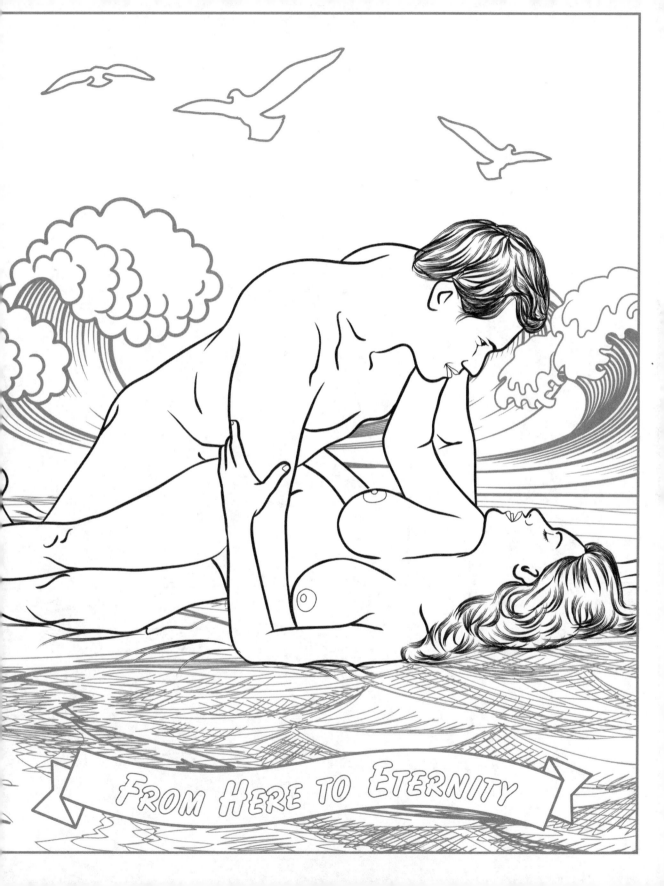

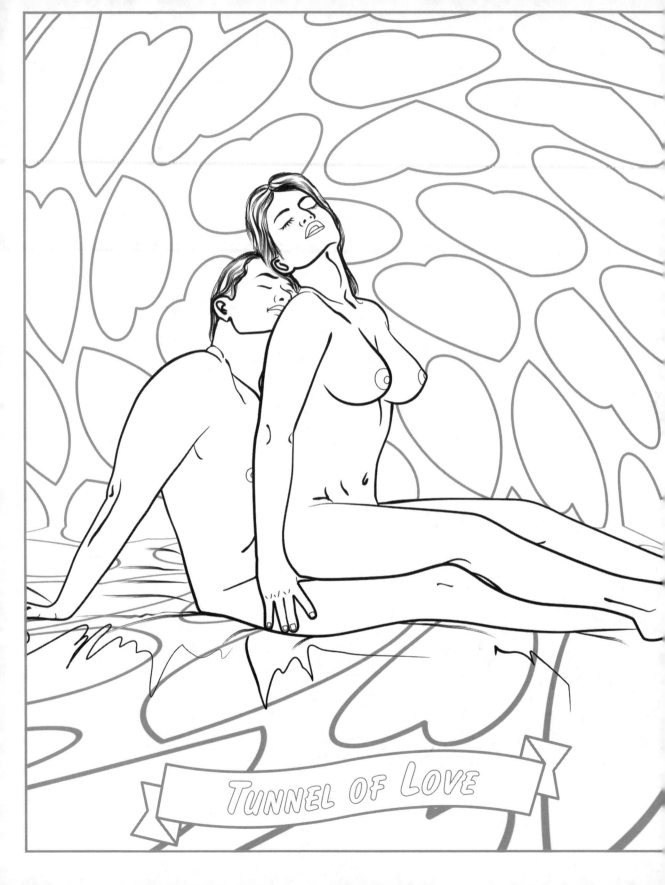

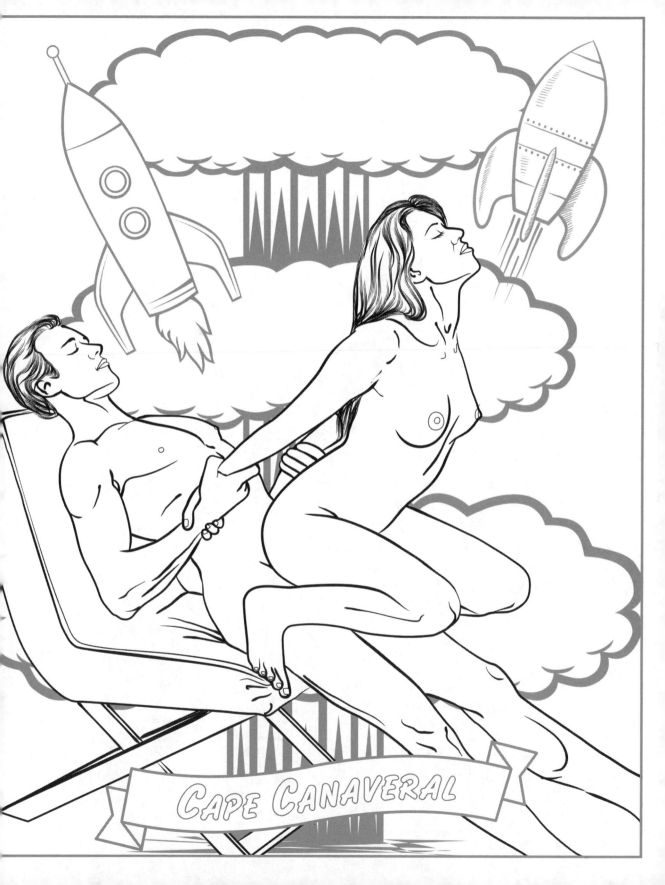

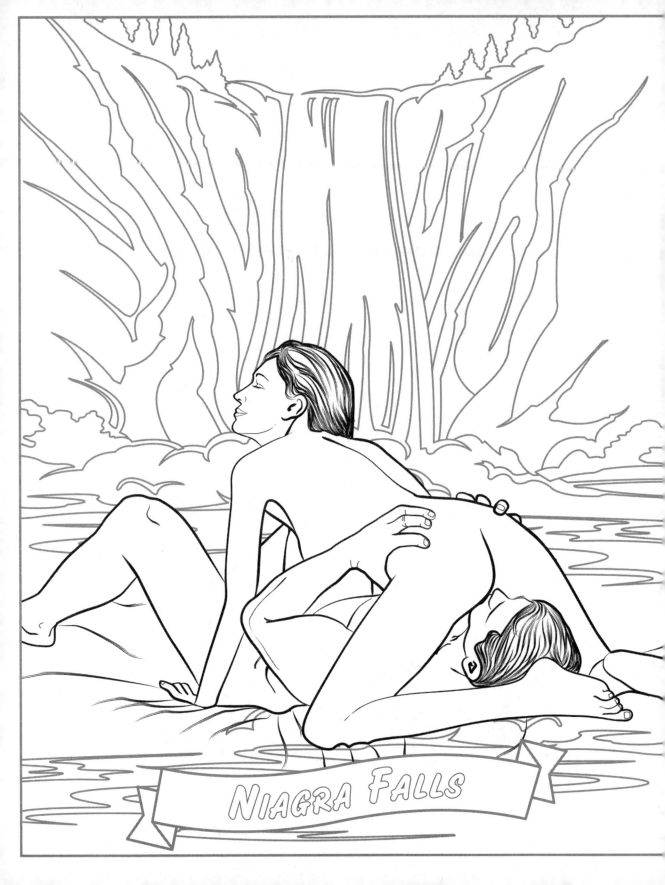

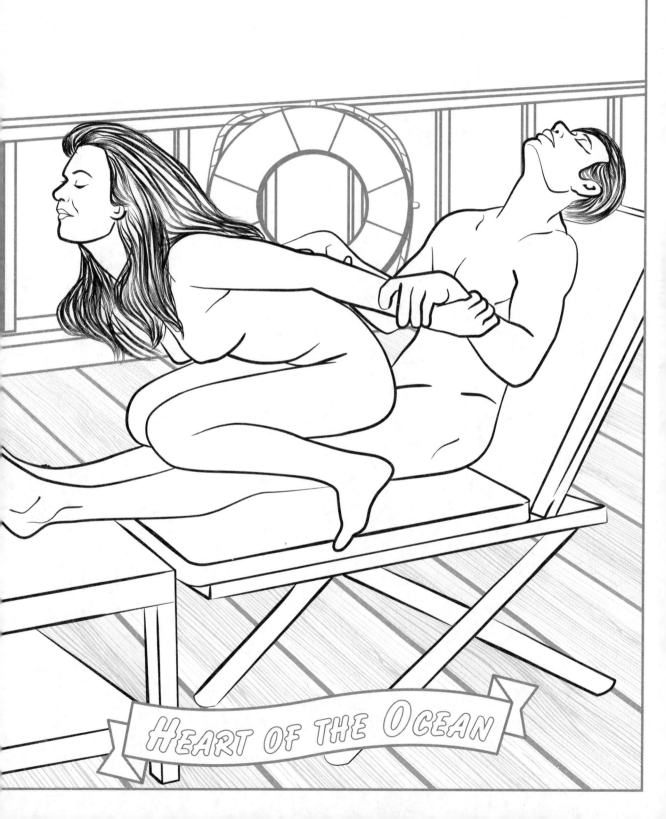

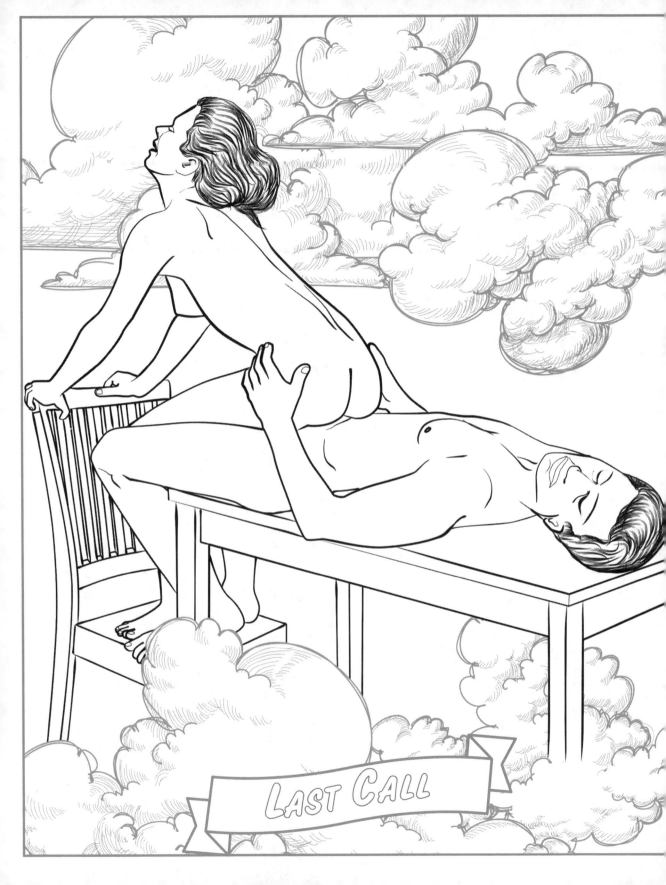

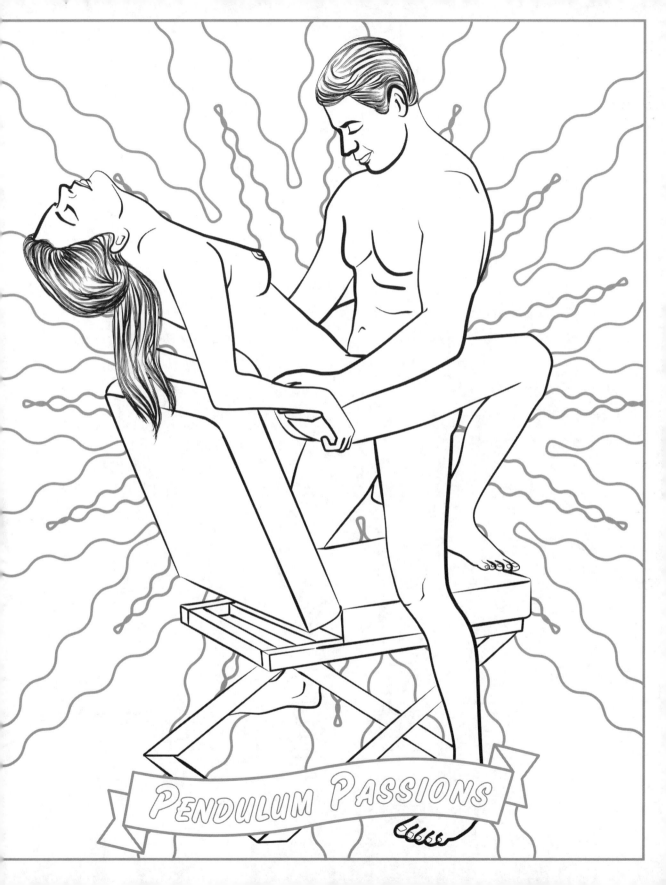

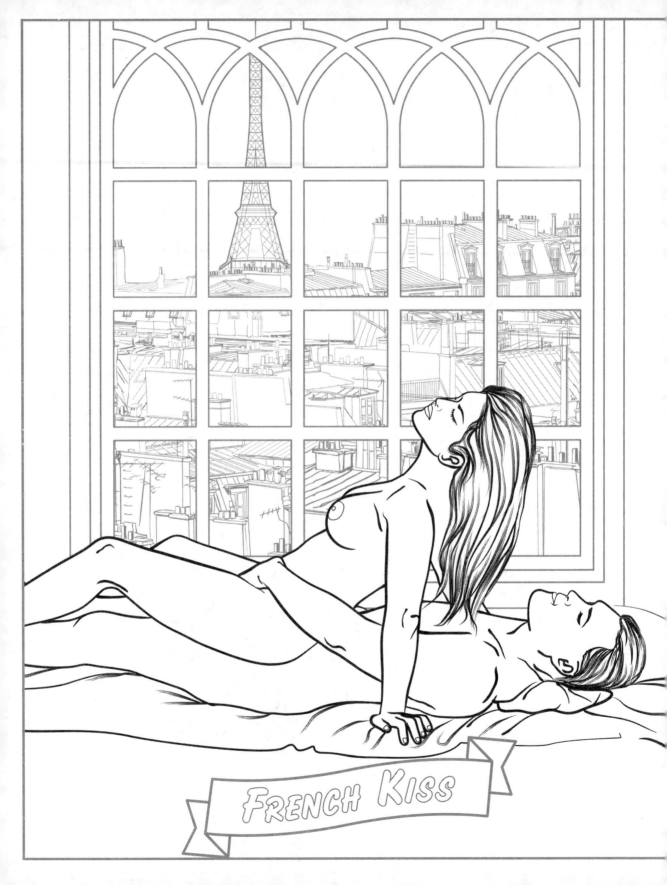

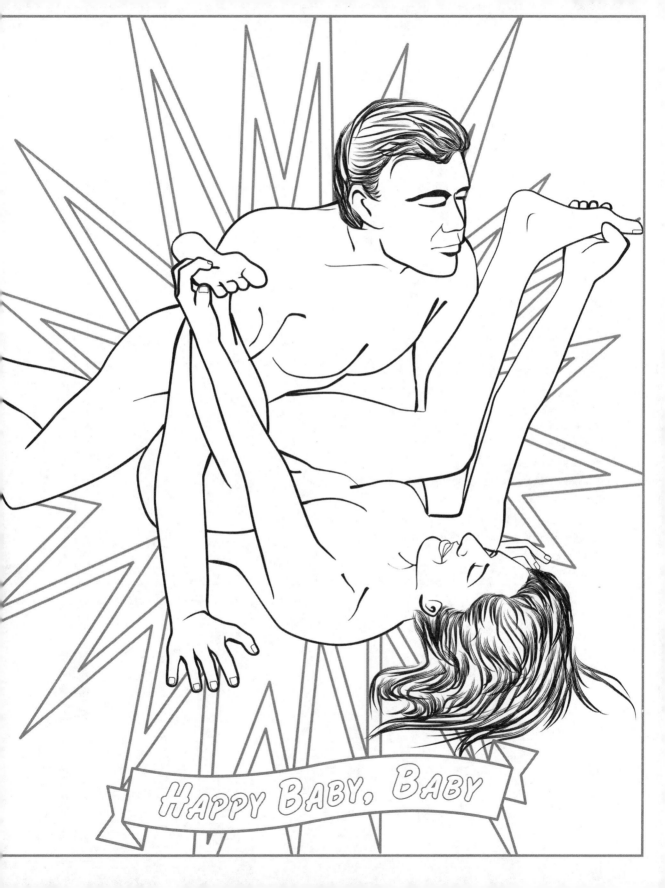

Image Credits

Illustrations are from shutterstock.com

You Stay Classy: wood grain © USBFCO
The Hasselhoff: © danussa
Lift and Carry: © Aleksandr Bryliaev
The Springboard: © freesoulproduction
Mahalo Nui Loa: © il67
The Cosmic Voyage: © Oksana Merzlyakova
Room with a View: © A-R-T
When in Rome: © VladisChern
The Last Unicorn: © Makarova Viktoria
Get into the Groove: ©Tashsat
Realm of Fantasies: © Uliana Gureeva
The Upstairs Downstairs: floor © A-R-T; fireplace © Canicula
What's for Dinner: © GLYPHstock
This Seems Natural: wood grain © USBFCO
Side Saddle: © Blue67design
Three Degrees to Nirvana: © krishnasomya
Peek-a-Boo: © Curly Pat
Opening the Lotus: © Shumo4ka
The Special Purpose: © freesoulproduction
The Springboard: © Feliks Kogan
The Pot of Gold: © Luisa Venturoli
Flight of Doves: © Danussa
The Mermaid: © ShineArt09
Anchor Light: porthole © vso
The Deck Chair: wood grain © USBFCO
The Bass Trombone: © Ozerina Anna

The Right to Remain Sexy: © Tatiana Kasyanova
Sabado Tarde: window © Valik-Novik; floor © Rodin Anton
Levitation Zen: © Krishnasomya
Marco Polo: wall © USBFCO; window frame © Elena Terletskaya; window blinds © metrue
The Spin Cycle: dryer © grmarc; laundry basket © Andre Adams
The Undertow: © il67
Playing Koi: © Christopher Brewer
Panamanian Fur: © karakotsya
Seven Senses © Roman Ya
Tender Loving Care: © Rostizna
The Longshoreman: © kalomirael
Deep Sea Diver: © Robert Adrian Hillman
Cancun Hammocks: © Danussa
Wild Stallion: left horse © insima; right horse © LVJONOK
Chin Music: © Roman Ya
Kissing the Rosebud: © POLINA 21
From Here to Eternity: waves © il67; water © danussa
Cape Canaveral: left rocket © Tribalium; right rocket © LHF Graphics
Niagara Falls: © SlipFloat
Heart of the Ocean: life preserver © Miguel Angel Salinas; wood grain © USBFCO
Last Call: © danussa
French Kiss: Paris © isaxar